SURVIVAL SWIMMING

SWIMMING TRAINING FOR ESCAPE AND SURVIVAL

SAM FURY

Illustrated by
YOPI MUHAMAD

Copyright SF Nonfiction Books © 2018
Updated 2020

www.SFNonfictionBooks.com

All Rights Reserved
No part of this document may be reproduced without written consent from the author.

WARNINGS AND DISCLAIMERS

The information in this publication is made public for reference only.

Neither the author, publisher, nor anyone else involved in the production of this publication is responsible for how the reader uses the information or the result of his/her actions.

CONTENTS

Introduction   1
General Water Safety   3

EFFICIENT SWIMMING

TREADING WATER
Sculling   9
Eggbeater Kick (Rotary Kick)   11
Treading Water   12

SWIMMING QUICKLY
Entry and Initial Propulsion   15
Underwater Fly-Kick   23
Freestyle   27

SWIMMING LONG DISTANCES
Survival Backstroke   39
Combat Sidestroke   41

SWIMMING LONG DISTANCES UNDERWATER
Safety   49
Stage One: Dry-Land Breath-Holding   50
Stage Two: Static Underwater Breath-Holding   52
Stage Three: Static Apnea Training   53
Stage Four: Efficient Stroke   56
Stage Five: 50m Swim   58

WATER SAFETY, SELF-RESCUE, AND SURVIVAL

Protective Clothing   61
Safe Entry Techniques   64
Survival Swimming Styles   69

Waves	71
Tides and Currents	74
Obstructions	77
Self-Rescue Bowline	85
Improvised Flotation Aids	86
Cold Water Survival	90
Flood	94
Swimming When Restrained	95
Survival at Sea	96

RIVER CROSSINGS

Choosing Where to Cross	103
Waterproofing Your Pack	104
Wading	105
Rope Crossings	109
Building an Improvised Raft	114
Swimming Across	119
Other Bodies of Water	121

WATER RESCUE

When You See Someone in Trouble	125
Situational Assessment	126

LAND-BASED RESCUES

General Land-Based Rescues	131

WATER-BASED RESCUES

General Water-Based Rescues	135
Towing	137
Defense Against a Drowning Victim	142

ROPE RESCUES

Land-Based Rope Rescues	149
Swimming Rope Rescues	154

References	157
About the Survival Fitness Plan	158
About Sam Fury	159

GET THE SURVIVAL FITNESS PLAN APP

It's like having Sam Fury as a personal coach to train you in the Survival Fitness Plan whenever you want!

Download it FREE at:

https://www.survivalfitnessplan.com/app

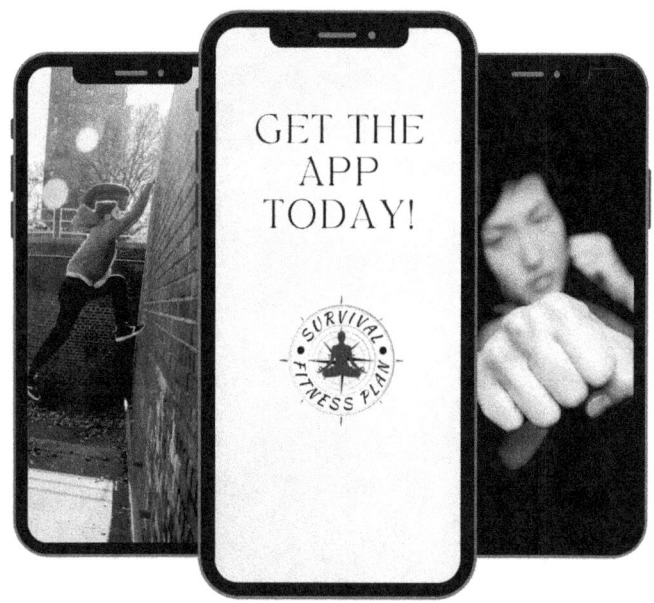

WWW.SURVIVALFITNESSPLAN.COM/APP

INTRODUCTION

Being in/near water is dangerous for humans. We cannot breathe underwater and swimming isn't instinctive. We must learn.

Even when we know how to swim, it's not a failsafe against drowning. This is especially true in open water, where there are many variables that can take us by surprise (weather, animals, riptides, etc.). But these dangers shouldn't stop you from swim training. In fact, they're even more of a reason to learn what's in this manual.

This book assumes you already know basic swimming strokes and techniques. It's a three-part manual:

Efficient Swimming

This section has techniques and training methods for improving your ability in swimming:

- Fast
- Long distance
- Underwater (speed and distance)

Water Safety, Self-Rescue, and Survival

Being near water has its inherent dangers, and being on open water has even more. This section has information about the different dangers in various forms of open water. It explains what to do when you're faced with these dangers, covering self-rescue and survival in solo and group scenarios. In this manual, the term "open water" refers to any natural body of water, such as an ocean, lake, or river.

Water Rescue

This section covers essential water rescue skills in both pools and open water.

Most of the information in this section draws on professional lifeguarding techniques, but it is NOT a replacement for professional lifeguard training! It's for emergency situations where no lifeguards are present—for example, when you're hosting a gathering near a lake or pool.

GENERAL WATER SAFETY

The activities in this manual can be dangerous if you do not take the proper precautions. Important note: Whenever possible, learn new techniques in calm waters (such as a pool). Only when you are confident should you practice them in open water. Always follow the water safety guidelines in this section and others:

- The best way to ensure safety is to avoid the danger in the first place. If total avoidance is not an option, the next best thing is to seek out local knowledge. Ask lifeguards, local surfers, paddlers, fishermen, etc. If you can, scout an environment out yourself, as circumstances may change.
- Always have a safety person, such as a training partner or a lifeguard, present.
- Protect yourself from the sun with appropriate clothing and sunscreen.
- Stay hydrated.
- Keep warm. This is covered in detail in part 2 of this manual.
- Don't go near water under the influence of drugs or alcohol.
- It's good to push yourself to improve, but be careful not to push yourself too much. This is especially true on open water.
- Have the correct safety and rescue equipment nearby, and know how to use it.
- Train only in waters and conditions you know to be safe. Look for signs and flags for the information you need, and if you are unsure, ask the lifeguards. Don't swim when the red flag is flying.
- Watch out for other people doing recreational activities, such as surfing or motorsports. Usually, they will have separate designated areas from swimmers.
- Never run or dive into unknown water. In open water, you must always check as conditions can change.

- If you get into trouble, stay calm and raise your arm to signal for help.
- Always wear a life vest when in a boat or any uncontrolled environment. Zip it up! A loose vest can get caught on many things.
- Tell someone who isn't going with you where you'll be training and when you expect to be back.
- Take care near the edge of any water body whether it be a pool, river, etc.
- Learn about the different characteristics of various water bodies before training in them.
- Enter and exit the water in a safe manner using designated entry and exit points, like ladders. Use your hands and feet, and take your time.

EFFICIENT SWIMMING

This section has techniques and training methods for improving your ability in swimming:

- Quickly
- Long distances
- Underwater (speed and distance)

TREADING WATER

Treading water is the most energy-efficient way to stay in one spot. Learn to do so before doing any other water-based training. This is so that if you need to, you can tread water until you either create a plan for self-rescue or help arrives. When you're first learning, tread in shallow water and with a lifeguard present. Progress to deep water when you're confident.

While you're treading water, your body is vertical in the water and your head is above the surface. Your arms and legs work to keep you afloat. Torso movement is minimal.

There are a few ways to tread water. The following method is a little harder to get the hang of, but it's the most energy efficient. It combines vertical sculling with your arms and the eggbeater kick.

SCULLING

To scull, move your arms back and forth in the water, not up and down. Turn your palms in the direction that your arms are moving. Angle your thumbs up a little on the way in, and your pinky fingers up a little on the way out. Keep your back straight. Don't lean forward or backward.

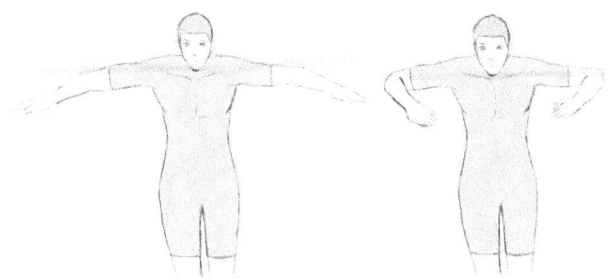

Vary the width of your stroke. Sometimes your hands should remain far apart, and sometimes they should almost come together.

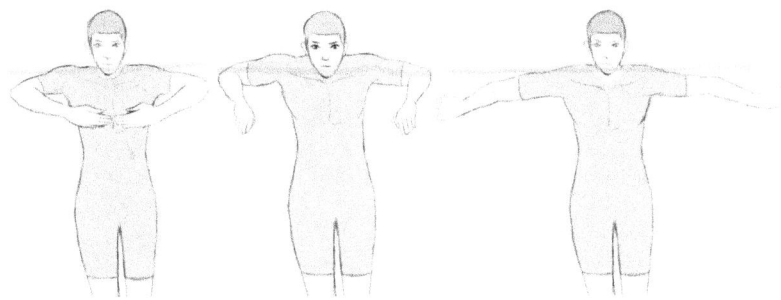

You can start by practicing this in shallow water. Find a depth where you can keep your head above water while you kneel. Begin the sculling action with your hands. Do it forcefully enough to raise your knees off the bottom.

When you're ready, move into deeper water. Place your feet directly underneath you, toes pointing straight down.

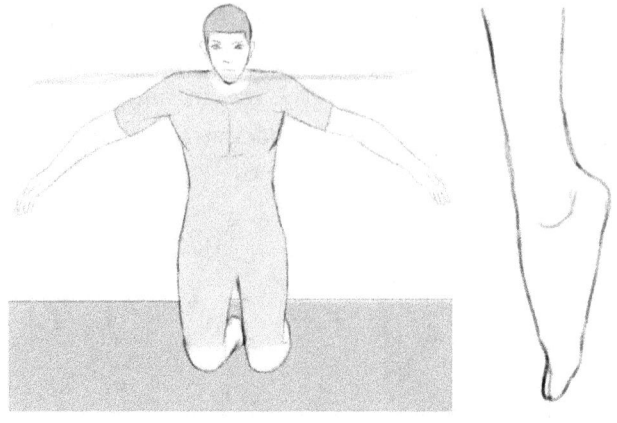

EGGBEATER KICK (ROTARY KICK)

The egg-beater kick can be tricky to learn, but it's worth going through the trouble. In comparison to the alternatives (such as the flutter kick), it's the most energy efficient.

Move your legs like an eggbeater, rotating each one in a different direction. It's like a breaststroke kick done one leg at a time. When one leg kicks out, the other should be coming in.

To begin learning the egg-beater kick, sit on the edge of a chair on dry land. Sit up straight and move only your right leg in a counter-clockwise circle. Next, move only your left leg in a clockwise circle. When you're ready, join these two leg movements together. As your right leg goes out, your left leg should come in, and vice versa.

Once you have the coordination, practice the egg-beater kick in the water. Lift your toes as you press down, so that your flat foot pushes down on the water, helping to propel you up. Point your toes as you bring your foot up, so that you have less resistance. Do not extend your legs completely. If they straighten out, you'll lose your upwards propulsion.

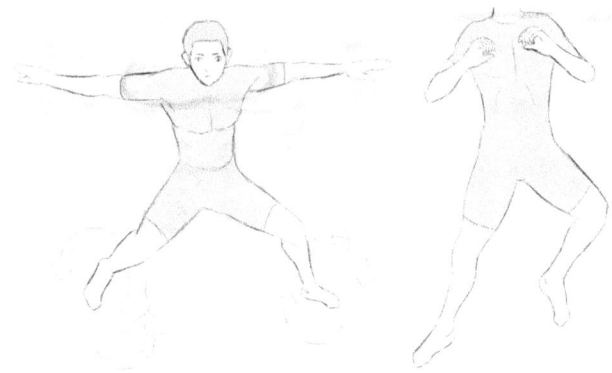

TREADING WATER

Once you're proficient at sculling and the eggbeater kick you can stay afloat by doing ONLY one or the other. You can perform tasks with your hands while staying afloat in one spot, and/or you can stay afloat in case of a leg injury.

By putting the two actions together, you'll conserve energy in both your arms and legs. This is ideal in a survival situation when you need to stay in one spot for long periods of time.

When treading water, stay calm and slow down your breathing. This will maximize your energy conservation.

Related Chapters:

- Eggbeater Kick (Rotary Kick)

SWIMMING QUICKLY

You will need to swim fast in emergency situations such as rescue or escape. Race swimming techniques are a base for this that you can then adapt for use in emergency situations.

There are three basic elements to consider when your goal is to swim quickly.

1. Entry and/or initial propulsion
2. Underwater swim
3. Surface swimming

Your initial propulsion is usually achieved by a dive entry or by pushing off something. Once you have your initial propulsion, you want to swim as fast and for as long as you can underwater. Use the fly-kick (either dolphin or fish tale). Swimming underwater is faster than surface swimming due to there being less resistance. When speed is your goal, swim underwater for as long as possible.

Once you need to surface for air, use freestyle (a.k.a. over-arm, front-crawl), since it's the fastest surface-swimming stroke.

It's assumed that you already know the basics of the three elements above. Now, we'll concentrate on improving the two factors needed to maximize speed for each element:

- Decreasing drag.
- Improving propulsion.

ENTRY AND INITIAL PROPULSION

You can use different entry and/or initial propulsion techniques depending on the situation. These techniques include:

- The push-off and streamlined position.
- The shallow dive.
- The dolphin dive.
- The deep-water floating start.
- The flip turn and push-off.

When speed is your primary goal, all these actions will lead into the underwater fly-kick.

Note: When you need to enter unknown waters, use the safe entry techniques described in part 2 of this manual. Opting for a safer entry technique may slow you down, but you won't be very fast at swimming if you get injured. Safety first, always.

Push-off and Streamlined Position

For the greatest speed when you're pushing off the edge, drop one to three feet below the water. When you're doing a flip turn, this will be automatic.

The best position for your legs/feet is shoulder width apart and with a bend in your knees. Push hard off the edge with strong legs and a tight core.

When you push off, your body must be as streamlined as possible. Become a straight arrow, stretching your body from your toes to your fingertips.

Place the palm of one hand on the back of the other. Wrap your upper hand's pinky and thumb around your lower hand, and then raise both hands over your head. Point your fingers in the direction you are going. Straighten your arms. Tuck them behind your head and squeeze your shoulder blades together. Another method is to squeeze your ears between your biceps.

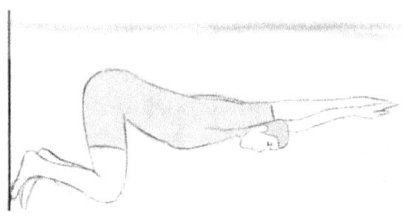

Keep your head down (swimming downhill), with the top of it pointing in the direction you want to go. Point your feet and turn your toes in towards each other a little (pigeon-toed). Keep your chin tucked and use a smooth exhale in whatever way is most comfortable for you.

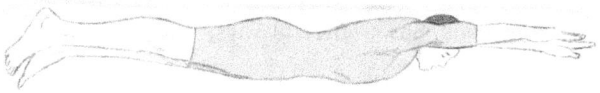

Maintain this streamline position as you push off the wall. Start the underwater fly-kick to maintain momentum underwater before surfacing into freestyle.

Note: Being on your side (as opposed to facing down) creates less resistance and may allow you to gain some speed. You should experiment with this.

Shallow Dive

Diving will give you the most propulsion, but is also the most dangerous entry method. **If you're unsure of the water depth and/or what lies below the surface, DO NOT DIVE!**

In an emergency, you may be pretty sure it's safe to dive, but not have the time for a thorough assessment. In this case, use the shallow dive. A shallow dive is one in which you arc into the water hands first while you adopt the streamlined position.

When you're starting to perfect your dive, do so from a stationary position. Place your lead (strongest) leg on the edge of the water (poolside, for example), with your toes a little over the edge. Your rear foot should be flat on the ground. Balance your weight evenly on both feet. Place your arms above your head in the streamlined position, with your chin tucked to your chest.

Push off with your lead foot so you get some distance. Arc over as you push and adopt the streamlined position as you enter the water.

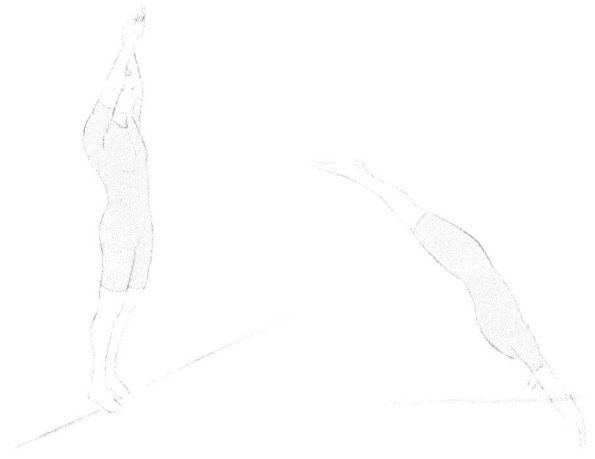

Once you are in the water, hold your head up and arch your back. This will steer your body up away from the bottom.

The more you arch, the more speed you will lose. You have to compromise depending on the water depth. Remember that you will be faster streamlining a couple of feet below the surface.

Note: Do not look/arch up before you are in the water. You will lose speed and may get injured.

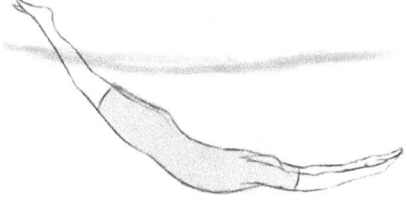

When you're ready, try diving from a walking and then a running start. In these cases, your arms will start by your sides. Once you leap off the edge, adopt the correct position so you can enter the water using the same basic form.

Dolphin Dive

Dolphin dives are useful when running into the water from a beach. They'll allow you to overcome waist/chest deep water as fast as possible. To preserve your forward momentum, run until the water is knee or waist high, and then use a dolphin dive.

As you run in, look out for obstacles in the terrain, such as rocks or holes. Once you hit the water, lift your feet completely out of the water for as long as possible. This will decrease your drag time. Put your hands in the streamlined position and leap/arc over into a dive.

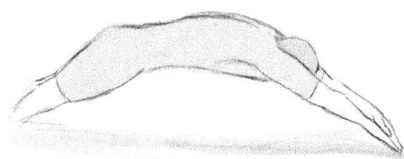

Don't dive too hard, or you might injure yourself, but dive deep enough to reach the sand on the bottom. Grab hold of the sand and lock your feet one in front of the other. Push forward off the ground into your next dolphin dive as fast as you can. Continue to dolphin dive in rapid succession until it's too deep to continue (about neck deep).

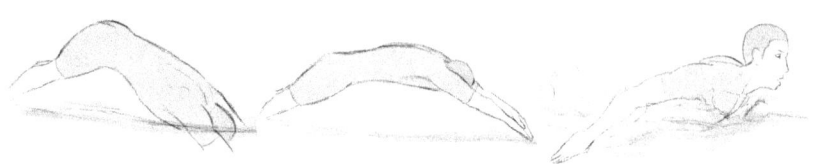

Do not look up while dolphin diving. As with the shallow dive, this is important for safety and speed.

If a wave is approaching, dolphin dive under it, grab the sand and stay under until the wave passes over you.

Once it's too deep to dolphin dive, transition into the underwater fly-kick.

You can also use the dolphin dive to come back into shore. Swim until it's shallow enough to dolphin dive, then continue to dolphin dive until you can run out.

Floating Start

Use a floating start from a floating/treading position when you have nothing to push off. The key for this is to use an explosive initial kick (such as a side scissor kick) and then go straight into freestyle. If you know that you will need a floating start, get as close to the freestyle position as possible.

Adopt a horizontal position. Place your dominant hand in front, ready to pull back into your first stroke. Have your other arm in a half-stroke position. Your heels should be close to the surface of the water. Tread water in this position.

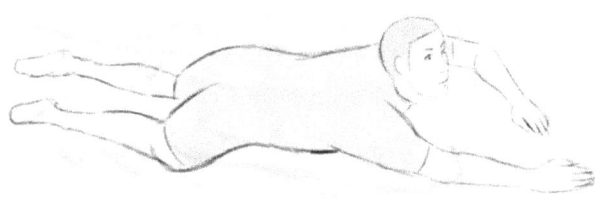

When it's time to swim, kick hard as you pull with your first stroke and transition into normal freestyle.

Flip Turns

Flip turns are often identified with swimming races in a pool. Having to turn in the water in an emergency is not likely, but it is possible. Knowing how to flip turn will make it much faster for you to do this.

First, learn the flip turn without having to push off the wall. In an emergency, this is most likely the style you will use.

The main flip part of the flip turn is actually only a half-flip. Start by swimming on your stomach (freestyle, for example). As your arm enters the water for the turn, start a half-flip by tucking your chin and doing a small dolphin kick. At the same time, move your hands to your sides. Breathe out through your nose to prevent any water getting up it.

Continue the half-flip by tucking your knees towards your eyes and your feet to your bum. At the same time, push down with the palms of your hands to get your feet over your head. Keep your elbows close to your body while doing this.

As you complete the half-flip, bring your arms into the streamlined position. You are now pointing in your new travel direction.

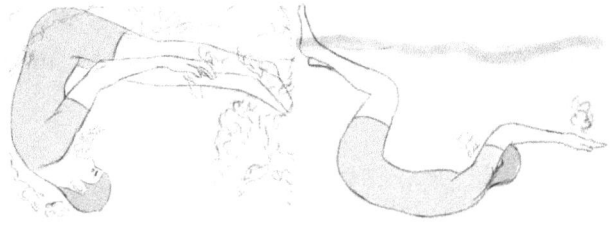

Roll onto your stomach by twisting your hands a little and looking in the direction you want to rotate. Don't turn your head; just move your eyes.

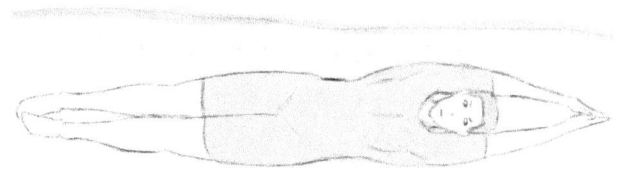

Use an explosive kick and arm pull to set you off in your new direction like you would in a floating start.

Note: Don't try to look where you are going during the flip. It will slow you down and mess up your coordination. Look at your knees instead.

To turn and push off a wall (such as in a pool swimming race) speed up (kick harder) when you are about five meters away from the wall. Ensure you have enough air to make the turn, but don't take a breath before it, as you'll slow down.

Once you are a bit more than an arm's length away from the wall, do the turn as normal. Push off the wall as described before (Push-off/Streamlined Position). The difference is that you'll be face up when you do the push-off, with your toes pointing up.

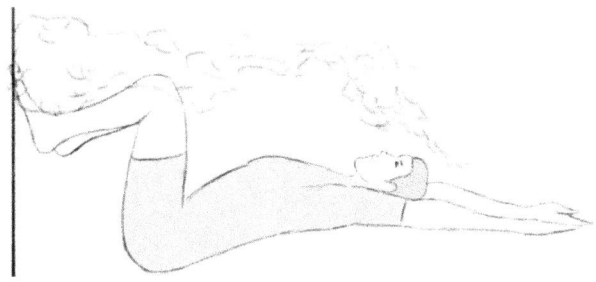

Once you push off, start to turn onto your stomach and then do underwater fly-kicks. You may wish to start to fly-kick before (whilst on your back), and/or during your turn. Experiment to discover what you prefer/works best for you. Continue to fly-kick until you need to start surface swimming.

Once you can do the basic turn and push off, work on perfecting your distance in relation to the wall. Land on your feet, with your knees bent close to 90° and your hips bent close to 110°.

Related Chapters:

- Underwater Fly-Kick
- Freestyle
- Safe Entry Techniques

UNDERWATER FLY-KICK

When you know how to do it, swimming underwater is faster than swimming on the surface. When you want to go fast, swim underwater for as long as you can.

The fastest way to swim underwater is using the underwater fly-kick. There are two main ways to do the underwater fly-kick: the dolphin kick and the fish kick. If you're good at it, the fish kick is faster than the dolphin kick, but in the Survival Fitness Plan (SFP), we focus on the dolphin kick because it is:

- Easier to master.
- Easier to control, especially in open water.
- Used in other strokes outlined in this manual.

Once you have the standard dolphin kick mastered, you may wish to progress to the fish kick. After your initial propulsion (e.g., dive or push-off), maintain your streamlined position. You want to maximize this glide phase before you start kicking.

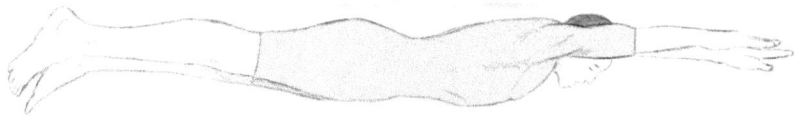

Just before you start to slow down, kick up and down with both feet/legs at the same time. Keep your upper body in the streamline position.

Bend your knees so that your kicks start and finish well in front of (or behind) your body, but do not kick from your knees. Use your core/hips to generate the power. To do this, suck in your stomach and squeeze your buttocks together.

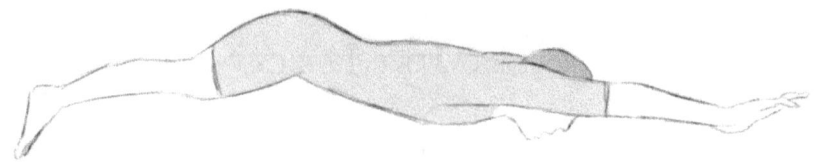

You must also snap your toes and ankle. It may help to think of your body as a whip. The power comes from your core (the handle), and your feet/toes are the tip of the whip, which snaps up and down. Kick fast and kick small. Ensure you also kick backward instead of only up and down. You want to push the water behind you. Your up and down kicks should be of equal force. Use the vertical kicking drill to develop your coordination and strength for this. The vertical kicking drill is in the Freestyle chapter.

When you start to surface, begin freestyle swimming.

Ankle Strength and Flexibility

Increasing your ankle strength and flexibility will improve your dolphin (and flutter) kick. Here are some exercises you can do:

Ankle rotations. Move your foot and ankle in a circle as large as possible without pain. Do 15–20 circles in each direction.

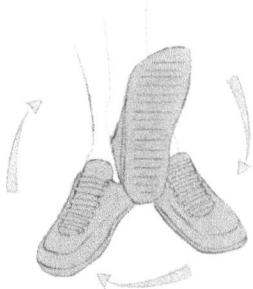

Ankle stretches. There are four levels of this exercise. Each increases in difficulty from the previous one. From a standing position, place the top of your toes on the ground a half step behind your other foot. Push down and forward into the ground. Sit on your heels, with your shins and the tops of your feet flat on the ground.

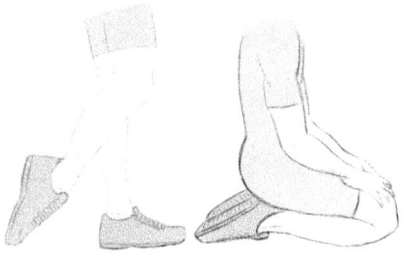

Lean back onto your hands to increase the stretch. Finally, put your hands up in the streamlined position and then lift your knees off the ground.

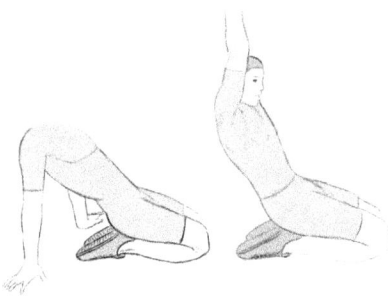

Ankle Inversion. From a standing position, roll one foot to the outside. Press the edge of your foot into the ground gently. Only do one foot at a time.

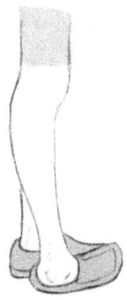

Related Chapters:

- Freestyle

FREESTYLE

This chapter assumes you already know the basic mechanics of swimming freestyle.

Freestyle (overarm) is the fastest way to surface-swim. By improving your technique, you will become faster and more energy efficient. There are a few different areas you can tweak. Practice in each individual area, and then put them all together when you're ready.

Balance

Being balanced in the water will make you more streamlined and so will increase your speed. Maintain a position that is as close to horizontal as possible.

Except when taking a breath, keep your head down and your neck relaxed. Imagine you have a blowhole in the back of your neck that you have to keep open. Looking down (as opposed to forwards) will also help.

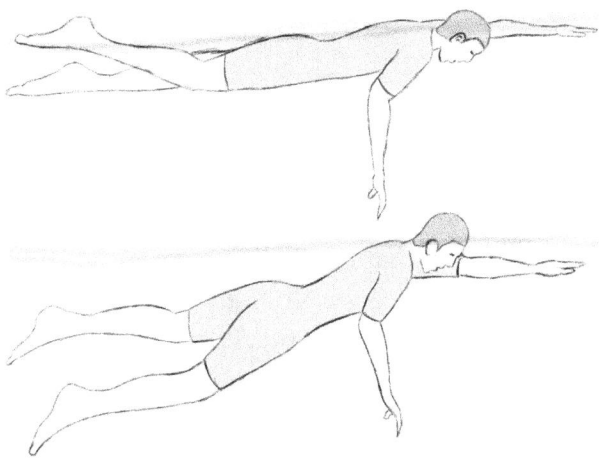

Breathing

Breathing while swimming (as opposed to holding your breath underwater) increases your stamina. Start blowing out as soon as you finish inhaling, and continue to do so until you take your next breath.

Experiment with breathing rhythms (take a breath every third or fifth stroke, for example) to see what works best for you. It may help to count your arm strokes (1, 2, 3, 4, breathe, for instance).

It is important to exhale completely before taking your next breath, so that you get rid of all the stale air. This increases your stamina and keeps you streamlined for longer. Every time you breathe, you break your streamline position.

Keep as close to your streamline position as possible while breathing. Do this by turning your head as opposed to lifting it out of the water. Your mouth only needs to be a little ways out of the water for you to inhale. Your eyeline should be no higher than the surface. If you're looking to the sky, you're turning your head way too much.

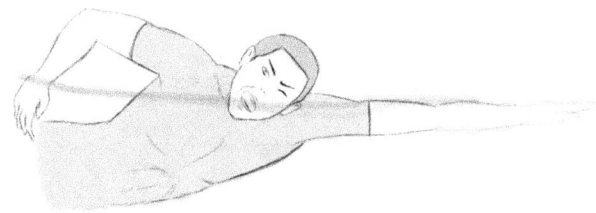

Breathing on alternate sides of your body (bilaterally) is a good habit. Always inhale through your mouth, but try to exhale most of the air through your nose. This is especially useful when you're turning/flipping, as it helps you avoid getting water up your nose.

Rolling

Roll from side to side with each arm stroke. This will engage your back muscles and improve propulsion. Engage your core as you do it.

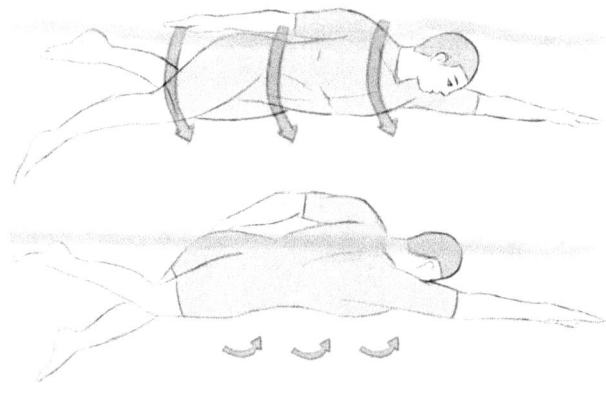

The following drill is good for getting used to floating on your sides.

Float flat on your back and do a light flutter kick for propulsion. Keep your body straight, with your arms at your sides. Apply downward pressure on the back of your head and on your shoulder blades, so that your hips and legs buoy up.

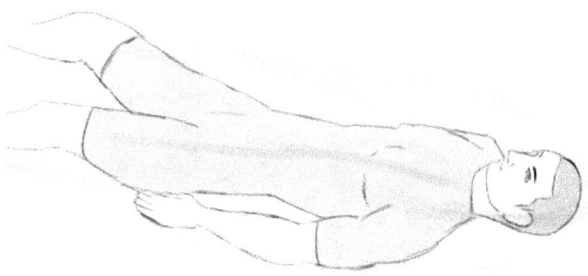

Once you feel balanced in this position, do the following:

- Roll onto your side so that your top arm and some of your top thigh clear the water.
- Do not move your while you roll on your side. Keep looking at the sky and roll your body as one.
- Continue to flutter kick.

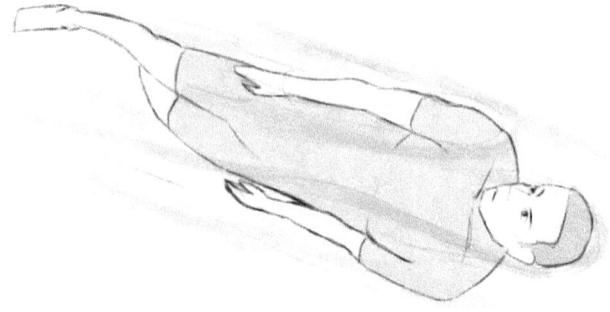

Roll as far as you're comfortable. A 45° body roll is good for most people.

Practice this on both sides of your body. Once you are comfortable with the above, advance by rolling to 90°, so that you face down.

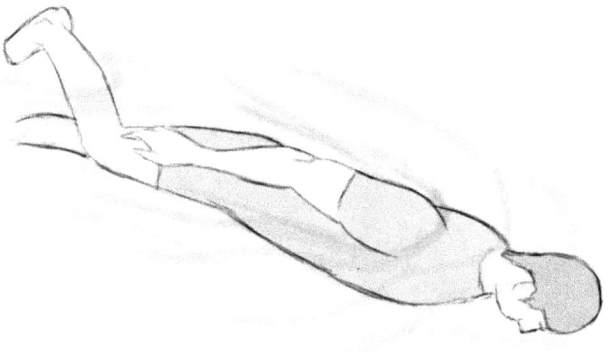

Keep flutter kicking, and keep balanced. Continue to roll in the same direction until you're in the 45° position, but on your opposite side. Remember to roll your whole body together. Don't lead with your head. When you're balanced, roll back the other way.

Arm Technique

The freestyle stroke is explained in four parts: the catch, pull, exit, and recovery. These four stages occur and repeat in the order listed.

There is a more advanced arm stroke known as the early vertical forearm position (EVF). It is harder to master, holds a greater risk of injury, and offers a minimal gain in speed. It's more for elite competitive swimmers. The following technique is like a non-extreme EVF.

THE CATCH is when your hand first enters the water.

Create a web with your hand by spreading your fingers apart a little, about 30% of the diameter of one finger. Maintain this spacing the whole time.

As you roll your body, stretch your arm out, with your palm faced down. Angle your fingertips downward a little and flex your wrist. Point your middle finger in the direction you'll travel. Place your hand in the water fingertips first. Ensure your arm/hand doesn't cross your centerline.

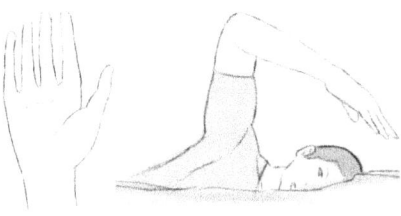

Once your hand is in the water, bend your elbow and press back on the water. Your forearm is in a near-vertical position. Don't push forward once your hand is in the water; it's better to go straight into the pull phase of the stroke. It may help to imagine your arm is moving over a big ball.

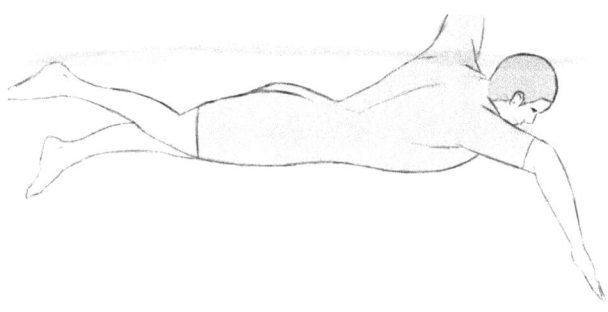

You can use finger paddles to help you perfect your catch. Wear them loosely. If you over-reach or have some other bad technique, the paddles will come off.

Another thing you can do is use a kickboard. Focus on making a good catch with only one arm. The kickboard will prevent you from reaching forward.

THE PULL is the movement of your arm in the water down the length of your body. After you make a good catch, your elbow will be in the "high" position. It will face the sky, while your palm faces to your rear. Keep this high elbow as you push the water behind you.

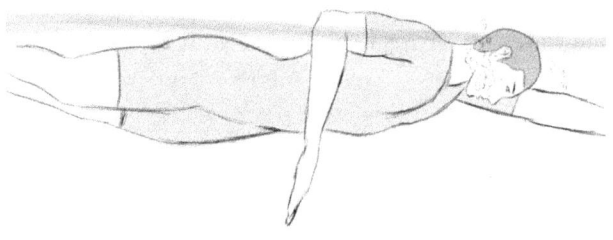

A good catch and pull is an easy, flowing feeling. You get great forward propulsion using your pecs and lats.

THE EXIT phase of your stroke is when your arm/hand leaves the water just past your hip.

It's important not to be too eager to bring your arm out of the water. Push beyond your hip as if you're trying to reach your knee, using the same press-up motion you would when exiting a pool using the wall. Do this push for the whole range of your pull, and as your thumb touches your thigh, flick the water out.

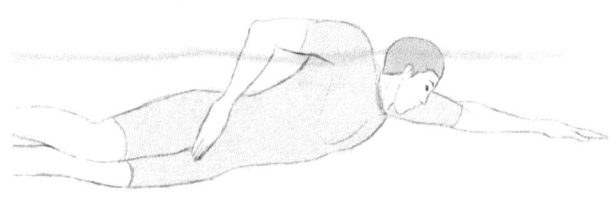

THE RECOVERY is the time when your arm is in the air. Your arm flicks out of the exit and then re-enters into the catch. It's best not to think about your recovery. Let it take its natural path. Your mental effort is better spent focusing on a great catch.

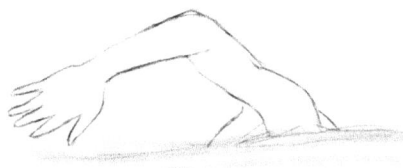

You can use stretch cords to practice all phases of your stroke on dry land. They're also useful for focusing on problem areas.

Efficient Kicking

A good kick is a compact one. It shouldn't be too low or break the water's surface. Don't disturb your natural alignment. Move your feet/legs independently of each other. Push one down as you pull the other up. Putting energy into both the up and down strokes is important.

Use short, quick kicks with your whole leg, starting at the hip. Keep your legs long and straight, but not rigid. Have a slight, natural bend in your knees. Point your toes behind you, but keep your ankles relaxed. Only the bottoms of your feet should meet the water's surface. Find a rhythm that's comfortable and stick with it. Around 15 kicks every 10 seconds is good.

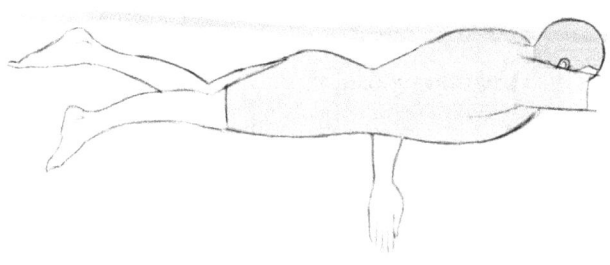

This vertical kicking drill will help to improve your flutter kick. It's also good for your dolphin kick. Do this drill in deep water, but make sure you are near something you can hold onto when you get tired.

Position yourself vertically in the water and do nothing but flutter kick to keep your mouth and nose above the surface. You will be kicking hard. Concentrate on the correct kicking technique, as described above. Begin with your arms underwater, and use a small sculling motion.

As you improve, try keeping your arms and hands tight against your body.

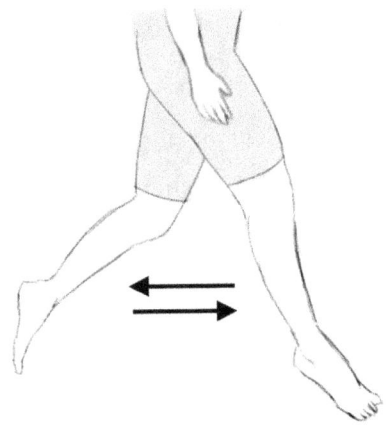

Advance further by raising your fingertips out of the water. Raise your arms higher and higher as you gain strength.

Transitioning from the Fly Kick to Freestyle

As you begin to surface, start to flutter kick and pull one of your arms down from the streamline position. Time the completion of your pull phase so that your arm exits the water as if you had been doing freestyle all along. This takes practice. Complete a few strokes before taking a breath, and then continue into freestyle as normal.

Additional Tips for Improvement

You can adapt most of these tips to all areas of swimming, and life in general.

- **Train regularly,** at least twice a week.
- **Compete against your times.** Notice what causes you to swim faster, and use what works best for you.
- **Identify and work on your weak points.**
- **Visualize someone chasing you.** Imagine you are being chased, then work on calming your mind and body and concentrate on swimming as fast as you can.
- **Get a professional swim coach.** Those of you who are having difficulties or want to get to the next level may benefit from guidance.

Related Chapters:

- Sculling

SWIMMING LONG DISTANCES

There are two strokes to learn for long-distance swimming: the survival backstroke and the combat sidestroke.

The survival backstroke, a.k.a. the elementary backstroke, is an easy to learn and is very energy efficient. It is for long-distance and/or survival situations, such as when waiting for rescue.

The combat side stroke (CSS) is an ultra-efficient variation of the sidestroke. It was developed by the Navy SEALS and is perfect for escape, evasion, and survival.

- It is efficient (fast yet energy conserving).
- You can do it with gear (like a backpack).
- Your body profile is lower (you'll be harder to see).
- It's excellent for swimming through the surf in open water.
- You can observe your surroundings as you swim, unlike with the survival backstroke.

SURVIVAL BACKSTROKE

This chapter assumes you know the basic mechanics of the survival backstroke.

The survival backstroke involves floating on your back as you propel yourself through the water. You use a simultaneous frog/breaststroke kick and a sculling motion with your hands. Your arms and legs move and come together at the same time.

The main goal of the survival backstroke is to conserve energy and reduce heat loss. To maximize energy conservation, do the survival backstroke very slowly. Take short strokes and glide for as long as possible. Only take the next stroke when you feel your legs dropping or you lose forward momentum.

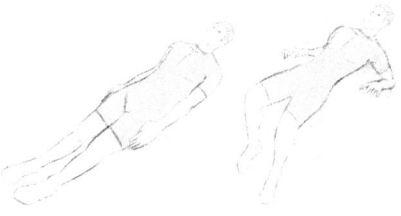

Taking short strokes minimizes heat loss from under your armpits and between your legs. Your arms should not extend beyond your shoulders. At the end of each stroke, bring your arms and legs together. Hold them close, but comfortably, against your body.

Use the survival backstroke is if an underwater explosion is likely. You will want to go faster so you can escape the blast, so make your strokes larger. Take your next stroke sooner than normal, but not too soon. Make the most out of your streamlined glide position while achieving the most speed.

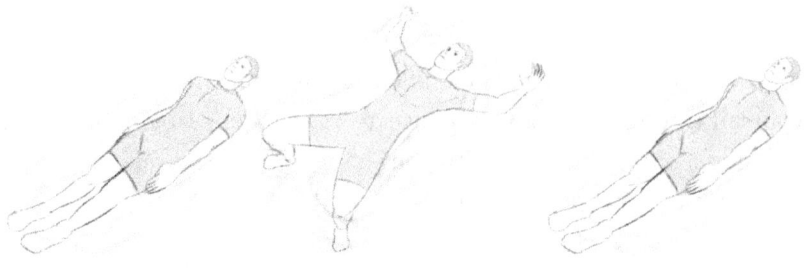

Related Chapters:

- Sculling

COMBAT SIDESTROKE

The combat sidestroke (CSS) is a mix of freestyle, breaststroke, and sidestroke. There are four basic stages to the CSS: the streamline position, two catch and pull movements, and the recovery. The recovery involves a scissor kick paired with a breaststroke-like arm movement.

Note: A lot of the terminology used in this chapter is explained in the Freestyle chapter.

Streamline Position

Get some initial propulsion. Adopt the streamline position, as explained in the Entry and Initial Propulsion chapter.

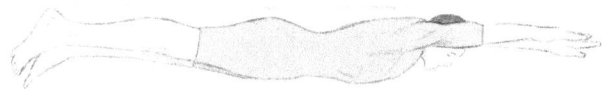

First Catch and Pull

Do your first catch by pressing the palm of your top hand down. If you are rolling to your right, then your right hand should be on top. Bend your arm at the elbow.

Make sure to keep your arm aligned at a downward angle. Your shoulder should be at the top, your elbow below that, then your wrist, and finally your fingers at the bottom. Doing this will maximize your first pull.

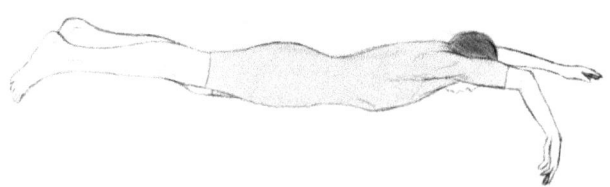

Continue the catch as you rotate onto your side. Your forearm should be positioned vertically, with your elbow above your wrist. Stay on your side until your recovery stage.

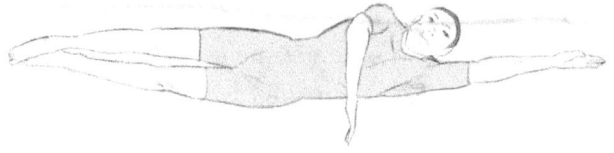

Flow into the pull by continuing the movement of your top arm until your hand is in line with your upper thigh. Your hand should follow your midline. Be careful not to raise your elbow too high.

At this stage, your arm should be almost fully extended. Do not let your hand come out of the water. Now is a good time to take a breath. When you exhale, do so slowly and steadily.

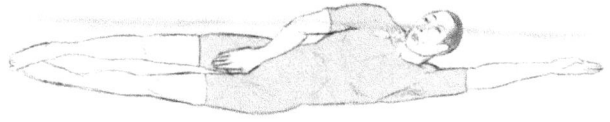

Second Catch and Pull

Start your second catch and pull with your other arm by sweeping it down. Your palm should face down and stay fixed in that position. As you sweep down, it will create resistance against the water, propelling you forward.

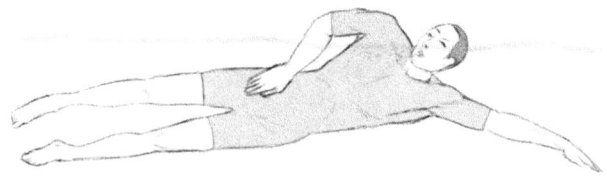

When your arm is vertical, your palm will be facing to your rear. Continue the arc of your bottom arm until your hand is on your thigh.

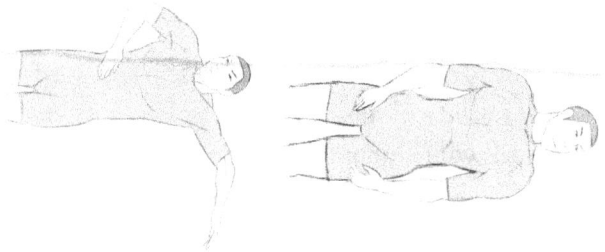

The catch, pull, and recovery of your lower arm is almost identical to a breaststroke motion.

Note: As you do the second pull you can either leave your head up breathing or look back down. If you tend to sink, you're better off looking back down.

Recovery

Start the recovery with a simultaneous scissor kick and arm movement.

Bring both your arms up through the centerline of your body, then back into the streamline position, like breaststroke. Keep your arms and hands underwater and as close to your body as possible. Move your arms forward past your face as you do the scissor kick. Finish in the streamline position.

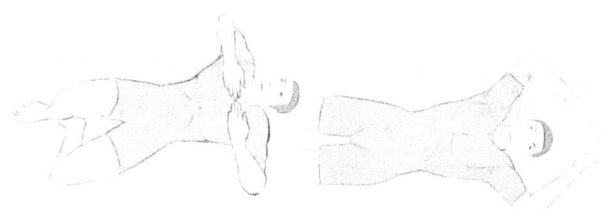

Scissor Kick

Do the scissor kick as you bring your arms forward. This helps with propulsion and corkscrews your body back into the streamline position.

Move your top leg forward and your bottom leg backward at the same time. Bring them back together in the streamline position. Keep your toes flexed towards your shin until you adopt that position.

Draw your top knee up so there is a 90° angle at your hip and knee. At the same time, bend your bottom leg back at the knee. Extend the lower part of your top leg in front of your torso as you kick your bottom leg back.

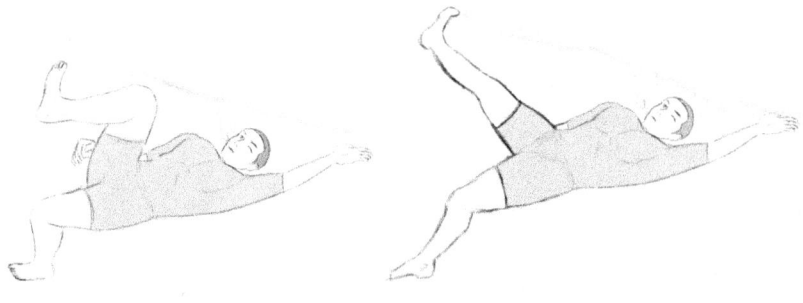

Point your toes once you have extended your legs, then draw them into the streamline position.

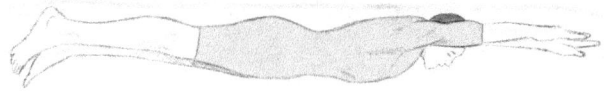

Slowly exhale as you glide in the streamline position. Be sure to get the most out of the glide before starting the next arm cycle.

If speed is more important, you can flutter kick before initiating your first pull again. You could also use the sprinter's CSS.

Sprinter's CSS

Use the sprinter's CSS when you need to go faster. The tradeoff is that you'll use more energy, since you'll have a greater stroke count over the same distance.

To do the sprinter's CSS, do a half-stroke on your second pull. Everything else will stay the same. From the start of the second pull, bring your arm down as normal, until it's almost at a right angle to your body. Instead of pulling it all the way to your thigh, scoop it up into your armpit.

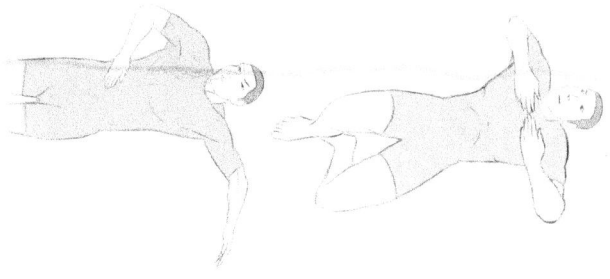

From here, push it forward into a full extension as normal.

Guide Stroke

Use the guide stroke to check your direction when using the CSS to swim a long distance. It uses a breaststroke-type movement for your arms and the dolphin kick for your legs.

Start in the streamline position. Push your palms out against the water to a position a little wider than your shoulders.

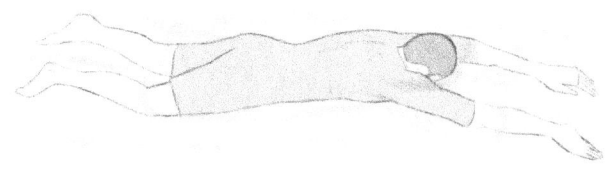

Press your palms against the water as you rotate your hands and lower arms into a vertical position. Your fingertips should point down, and your palms should be angled toward your chest.

Pull your palms towards your chest. This creates forward propulsion and allows you to raise your head above the surface. Now you can breathe and look around, but try not to lift your head too far out of the water, as this will cause your hips and legs to sink, and decrease your momentum.

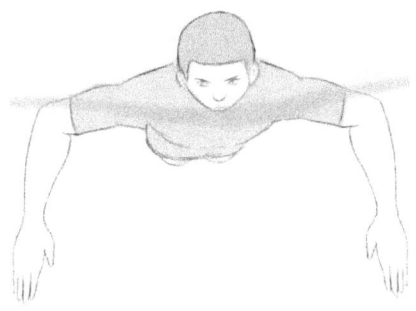

Move your arms back to the streamline position as you would with breaststroke. Keep them close to your body along your centerline.

As you recover your arms, use the downward motion of the dolphin kick. This helps with propulsion back into the streamline position. From here, you can continue into CSS or another guide stroke.

Note: For more instruction on the dolphin kick, see the underwater fly-kick chapter.

If you get disoriented, tread water until you figure out which direction you need to swim in.

Related Chapters:

- Entry and Initial Propulsion
- Underwater Fly-Kick
- Freestyle

SWIMMING LONG DISTANCES UNDERWATER

There are two major factors when it comes to swimming long distances underwater:

1. Efficient stroke.
2. Lung capacity (how long you can hold your breath).

This section offers a five stage-training plan. Use it to increase your ability to swim long distances underwater.

Important note: Depriving yourself of oxygen is dangerous. Safe training is paramount!

SAFETY

Here are some safety pointers to keep in mind when you're practicing to swim long distances underwater:

- Train with a partner, and not at the same time. Your friend must watch you so he can help if something goes wrong. If you must train alone, then at least make sure there is a lifeguard present.
- Stay in shallow water, especially to begin with.
- Never push yourself to beat your last time or distance. Only hold your breath for as long as is comfortable. Trying to beat your record will have an adverse effect anyway. You're much better off staying relaxed and seeing where you pop up.
- If you begin to panic at any moment, relax and surface.
- Listen to your body. If you get light-headed, your vision begins to fade, or you get any other abnormal sensation, surface immediately.
- Work on your lung capacity on dry land, and concentrate more on making efficient strokes when you're in the water.

STAGE ONE: DRY-LAND BREATH-HOLDING

Practice holding your breath for longer periods of time while you're on dry land.

In the Survival Fitness Plan, we use minimal preparation for breath-holding. This is so you know how far you can get in emergency situations. Breathe in, breathe out, breathe in, then go.

Take these breaths slowly, from deep within your diaphragm. This is to rid your lungs of low-quality air (CO_2).

You know you're using correct breathing if your belly, not your shoulders, is moving up and down. When your chest and shoulders move, it means you're breathing with only the top part of your lungs. This deeper breathing is also useful for recovery after a workout.

While doing the following, relax your muscles and remain as still and as calm as possible. Don't do any clock-watching, as it will make you anxious. The more relaxed and still you are, the less oxygen your body will consume.

Follow these detailed instructions for the inhale, exhale, inhale, sequence:

- Breathe in for a count of 5 seconds, hold for 1 second, then breathe out for a count of 10 seconds.
- When exhaling, push out every last drop of air, and push your tongue up against your teeth. This forms a valve which helps to control the release of air. Your breath should make a hissing sound as you exhale.
- Inhale slowly, to about 80–85% capacity. Start at the bottom, near your diaphragm, then up into your sternum, and finally into your chest.

- Hold your breath for as long as you can, and when you first start to feel the need to breathe, swallow a little spit. This helps to relax your breathing reflex.
- When you need to breathe out, let out little puffs of air at a time.
- When you're finished, push out as much air as possible to get rid of any extra carbon dioxide.

Don't try this sequence again until you get your body back to normal oxygen levels. Breathe steadily for at least five minutes, and don't do it more than three times in a single session. Only do one session a day.

After a few practice sessions, try adding in slow movements, such as walking. This will prepare your body to dive and swim with less air.

STAGE TWO: STATIC UNDERWATER BREATH-HOLDING

Stage two is the same as stage one, but underwater. The point of this stage is to get you comfortable holding your breath underwater.

Inhale, exhale fully, inhale to 80% capacity, then hold and submerge. Keep your mouth and nose closed while underwater. Use your fingers to hold your nose shut if you need to.

Stay relaxed, and resurface once you're near your limit. Blow out any extra air as you rise, so that you can take a fresh breath immediately.

STAGE THREE: STATIC APNEA TRAINING

In this stage, you will use static apnea training. This conditions your lungs and body to withstand the effects of prolonged breath-holding. This stage is ongoing. You can move on to stage 4 while doing it.

Important note: This is a dry land activity. DO NOT try it underwater!

There are two separate programs for static apnea training. One increases your CO_2 tolerance. The other increases the amount of oxygen your lungs can store.

Each program has its own training table. The recovery stage is when you can breathe normally for the allotted time. During the breath-hold stage, hold your breath for the allotted time. Only start O2 tolerance training once you can hold your breath for at least 90 seconds. You can do both CO_2 and O_2 sessions on the same day, but do not do them immediately after one another. Do one in the morning and one at night. Do not do more than one of each per day.

CO2 Tolerance

CO_2 tolerance training consists of a series of alternating breath-holds and rest periods. Your breathing time gets shorter, while the time you hold your breath holding stays the same. Start off with a breath-holding period that you're comfortable with. Try 50-70% of the maximum time you can hold it. Add 5 or 10 seconds each day.

The table below outlines one training session in which you recover and hold your breath eight times. Use the same breath hold time for each one. In your next training session (the following day), increase the time you hold your breath by 5 or 10 seconds.

#	Recovery	Breath Hold
1	2m 30s	50-70%
2	2m 15s	50-70%
3	2m	50-70%
4	1m 45s	50-70%
5	1m 30s	50-70%
6	1m 15s	50-70%
7	1m	50-70%
8	45s	50-70%

O2 Tolerance

In O2 tolerance training, your recovery period stays the same. Instead, you increase your breath holding.

Only start O2 tolerance training once you can hold your breath for at least 90 seconds.

This table shows one training session.

#	Recovery	Breath Hold
1	2m	50%
2	2m	55%
3	2m	60%
4	2m	65%
5	2m	70%
6	2m	75%
7	2m	80%
8	2m	85%

Additional Ways to Increase Your Breath-Holding Ability

There are some other things you can do to increase your breath-holding ability:

- Exercise often.
- Lose weight if you are overweight.
- Learn to play a wind or brass instrument.
- Take up singing.
- Don't do drugs, and especially avoid smoking!

Body Response Information

This is for informational purposes. DO NOT practice/experiment with it.

When you hold your breath for an extended period, your body goes through three response stages:

1. **Convulsions.** When you first get an urge to take a breath and you don't, you will have convulsions in your diaphragm. You can learn to fight through this, and if you do, you will gain a couple of minutes before you need to breathe.
2. **Spleen release.** If you fight through the convulsions your spleen responds by releasing oxygen-rich blood. Your body will calm down and you'll get a surge of energy. Use this energy to get somewhere that you can breathe!
3. **Blackout.** If you do not find fresh oxygen, you will black out. If you're underwater at the time, you'll drown.

STAGE FOUR: EFFICIENT STROKE

This teaches the technique for an efficient underwater stroke. The only aim is to learn the stroke. Don't try to break any underwater distance records. This stroke uses a combination of a modified breaststroke (for the arms) and the dolphin kick. Do it as one fluid motion. Start off in a streamlined glide and stay in it for as long as possible.

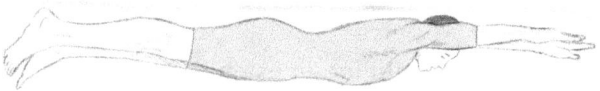

When you are almost to a complete stop, turn your palms out and separate your hands. Do the out-sweep of the breaststroke. Use webbed fingers, as described in the Freestyle chapter (under the heading Catch). Allow your legs to float up—the higher the better. Keep your head down.

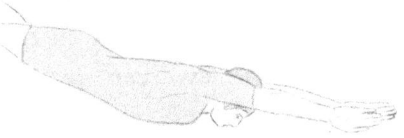

As you do the breaststroke arm movement, arch your body, extending your back and shoulders. You aim is to make your body like a spring that you'll snap down to propel you forward. Bring your arms and forearms into a vertical position, elbows facing up. Snap your arms and legs down together.

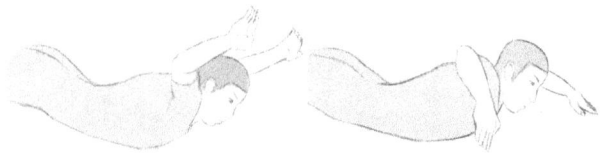

Do a dolphin kick and go into a double-armed pull stroke by pushing against the water down along your body. Remember your webbed fingers.

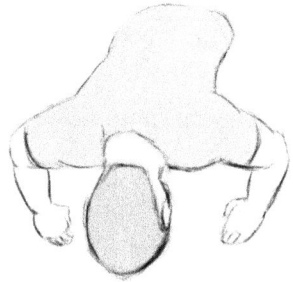

Keep your arms vertical for as long as you can and end in a streamline position with your arms by your sides. Glide in this position for as long as you can.

Do a standard breaststroke frog kick. At the same time, bring your hands back into the streamline glide you started in, with your arms/hands in front of you.

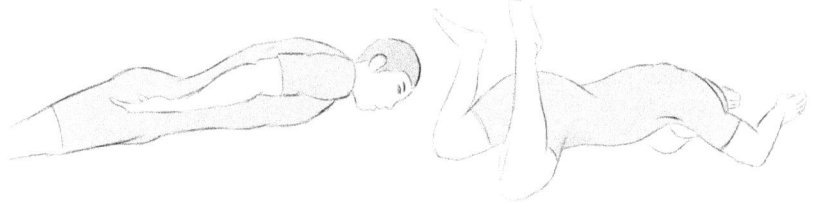

Repeat this sequence. When you start to run out of breath, go into your preferred surface stroke. CSS or freestyle is best.

Related Chapters:

- Freestyle

STAGE FIVE: 50M SWIM

Revisit the safety pointers from the start of this section.

Before attempting this final stage, you should be able to:

- Swim 25 meters underwater in under 30 seconds, using 5 strokes or less.
- Hold your breath for at least 90 seconds while walking on dry land.

The first part of stage five is building up your breath holding ability while moving on dry land. Hold your breath while doing SFP super-burpees for a minute. When you can do six in a minute, you're ready to attempt the 50-meter underwater swim.

You can learn about SFP super-burpees at:

www.SurvivalFitnessPlan.com/Daily-Conditioning-Workout/#Super_Burpees

Related Chapters:

- Safety

WATER SAFETY, SELF-RESCUE, AND SURVIVAL

Being near any body of water has its inherent dangers, and open water has even more. This section has information on the different dangers in various forms of open water. It explains what to do when faced with these dangers, covering self-rescue and survival in solo and group scenarios.

In this manual, the term "open water" refers to any natural body of water, such as an ocean, lake, or river.

PROTECTIVE CLOTHING

Protect yourself from cold and injuries with the appropriate clothing. Just because it's hot outside doesn't mean it will be warm in the water. It only takes a slight change in weather to take a situation from fun to dangerous.

- Wear the right clothing and use layers.
- Choose fabrics that provide warmth even when they're wet, not cotton or denim.
- In colder conditions, use a wetsuit.
- Once out of the water, put on warm clothes. Use clothing that blocks the wind, such as a poncho.

Layering

Layering means wearing several items of thin clothing as opposed to one or two thick ones. If you get too warm, you can strip one or two layers without losing all your protection. There are three basic layers: base, insulator, and outer.

Base layer. This first layer will reduce water flowing past your skin, and is also good for sun protection. You want a skin-tight, quick-drying material that will wick the water away. Rash vests are a good example. Polypropylene, polyester, and Lycra are good materials for your base layer.

Insulating Layer. The insulating layer keeps you warm when it gets colder. It should fit snugly, but not too tightly. Use materials that dry quickly. Unlined tracksuits work well, as do wool and fleece. It is important that the material be unlined; otherwise, it will hold air and water. A hooded top helps to prevent heat from escaping through your head. It also provides sun protection. Adjust the number of insulating layers you use depending on the temperature. In warmer climates, you may not even need one.

Outer Layer. Your outer layer should be a water- and windproof shell. Its purpose is to keep you warm and keep the elements, such as wind and rain, out, though you'll still get wet, either from perspiration or from being in the water. A rain jacket, an anorak, or a light nylon over-all works well. It should be large enough so you have good freedom of movement. This will also trap a warm layer of air inside it. It's important for the clothing in this layer to be windproof.

Other Clothing

Footwear. Footwear is especially important in unknown waters where your feet may get injured. Simple canvas shoes with drain holes work well. Wear ones that are easy to remove in case you get caught in rocks. Wearing socks as well provides insulation and prevents chafing.

Swimming in footwear, as with any clothing, will create extra drag. Experiment with it during training.

Goggles. Swimming goggles, or a mask, are not essential, but are useful if you want to see underwater. It's a good idea to always wear goggles in a chlorinated/chemical pool.

Poncho. A poncho is an excellent all-around piece of survival equipment. In water training, you'll use your poncho for some self-rescue exercises. It can also become an improvised shelter or emergency blanket (extra warmth) when you're not in the water.

Visibility

For your safety and, you want to be visible in the water. You want it to be easy for any water traffic and/or rescue services to spot you.

Maintenance

Always wash yourself and all your gear in fresh water after training in any water. This will keep everything in the best working condition for as long as possible. Rinsing your gear under a tap is not enough. Most of the bad stuff (salt or chemicals) won't get washed out. It's best to wear your gear in the shower or put it in the washing machine.

Restrictions

The more clothes you have on, the harder it will be to swim. Water-logged clothes will also make climbing out of the water harder. The best way to prepare is to simulate falling into the water while clothed, and then swimming to safety.

SAFE ENTRY TECHNIQUES

There are a variety of ways to enter the water. The methods described in this section focus on safety and are also used in rescue situations. Always enter shallow or unknown waters feet first. Unknown waters are those whose depth you're unsure of, and/or those you can't see into.

Wade Entry

When possible, the wade entry, or walking into the water very carefully, is the best way to enter unknown waters. Feel your way forward with your feet until the water is chest-deep, then start to swim.

Slide Entry

Use the slide entry for shallow or unknown waters with a steep-angled edge, such as a pool edge. It's also useful in crowded areas, since it's easier to control than other entry methods. The slide entry is very simple. Sit down with your feet/legs hanging down into (or above) the water. Use your hands to slide yourself into the water. In shallow waters, continue forward using the wade entry once your feet are firmly on the bottom.

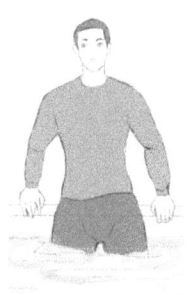

If speed is a factor and you plan to push off the wall once you're in the water, don't push too hard during the slide entry. If you're too far away from the edge, you won't be able to do a good push-off, which is what your initial propulsion comes from.

Step-off Entry

When you're entering shallow or unknown waters and you're too high for a slide entry, use the step-off. Step off your platform into the water. Keep your knees flexed and be ready to absorb any impact in case you hit the floor. You can then wade or swim, depending on the situation.

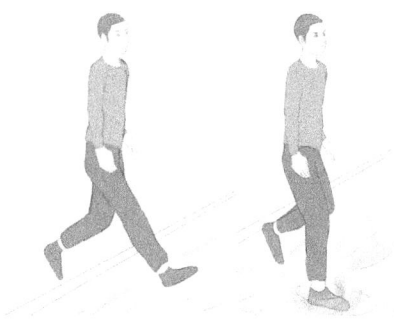

Stride Entry

Only use the stride entry when you know the water is at least 1.5 meters deep, and the slide entry is not appropriate.

One of the big advantages of the stride entry is that you keep your head above the water. This means you can keep your sight on something, such as a drowning victim.

Put your arms out to your sides and set one foot out in front of you. Plant your foot well so you don't slip. Keep looking at your target the whole time. Look up a little as you lean forward into the water. Slap your hands down as you hit the water. Looking up and slapping down helps to keep your head above the water.

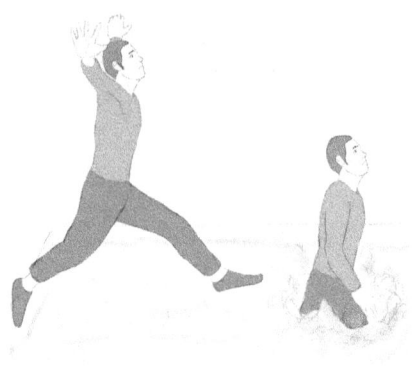

High-Level Entry

This is good to use when you have to enter the water from a height of 3+ meters. You must be sure that the water depth is appropriate for the height you are jumping from. Also ensure that your landing zone is long and wide enough.

Unlike all the previous entry methods, the high-level entry is not safe to do while you're carrying gear. If you have a backpack or anything else, throw it in before jumping. Consider wearing long clothing as it will help protect your body.

Take a large breath and jump away from the surface. You don't want to hit anything on the way down. Cross your ankles and place your hands in fists in front of your thighs. This puts your arms down and close to your body. Bend your knees a little.

Look straight ahead at the horizon and arch your back. Looking down or up will cause you to lean forward or back respectively. Arching your back will help keep you straight. You want to hit the water as close to straight up and down as possible. Allow your knees to flex once you do. This will help slow you down.

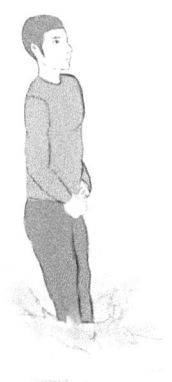

Height vs Water Depth

The higher your jumping-off platform, the deeper the water needs to be.

The best way to judge is if you have seen others do it, and even then you must be very careful.

Note: All these calculations are only approximate, so it is easy to do them in your head. The results are good enough to use.

Start with at least 2.5 meters (m) of water depth. If you're jumping from more than 1.5 m, you need to add an extra 0.6 m of depth for every 3 m increase in height.

A simple but effective way to calculate your height from the water is to drop something into it. Any solid object that won't catch air, like a rock, will work. Time how long it takes to hit the water.

Multiply that number by itself, and then multiply that answer by 16. That is, use the calculation $(x^2) \times 16$. This will give you the approximate height in feet. Multiply it by 0.3 to convert it into meters.

To calculate water depth, get a long stick (or something similar) and lower it in the water until it hits the bottom. Measure how much of it gets wet. This is easy in theory, but hard in practice.

Related Chapters:

- Safety

SURVIVAL SWIMMING STYLES

To successfully overcome obstacles in the water, you need to adjust your swimming style to the situation and what lies ahead.

The Defensive Position

In most cases, the best thing to do when experiencing trouble in the water is to tread water and signal for help. When you're in swift water, treading may not be practical, as the current will drag you away. In this case, the best thing to do is adopt the defensive position.

Get on your back with your feet up, so you can see your toes. Float downstream feet-first. This position will enable you to see the path ahead. Guide yourself through the safest route of passage. If you encounter any obstructions, absorb their impact with your legs. Keeping your feet up ensures they don't get caught in obstructions beneath the surface. Never try to stand up in river rapids that are deep enough for you to float in.

When you see an obstruction you want to avoid, angle your body so that your feet point towards the obstacle. Aim the top of your head towards your destination and use a modified sculling motion to get there.

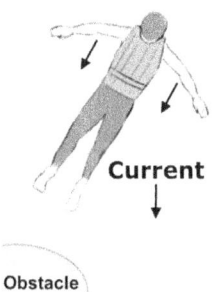

The Aggressive Position

If you see an opportunity to reach safety, you can use an aggressive position to get there, assuming the water is deep enough for you to do so. The aggressive position is doing freestyle while keeping your head out of the water.

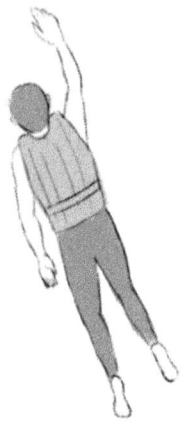

The aggressive position is very tiring, so reserve it for when you need short bursts of power. You could also use a breast or sidestroke. They will be slower, but will give you better visibility.

Related Chapters:

- Sculling
- Freestyle
- Obstructions

WAVES

If you're able to identify the types of waves, you can make the best decision about whether it's safe to swim in them or not. There are three basic types of waves to look for: spilling, plunging, and surging.

Spilling Waves

A spilling wave forms when the crest of the wave tumbles down its front. If the sandbank it breaks on is shallow, it will form a tube.

Spilling waves occur on ocean floors with a gradual slope. They are most common with onshore winds (winds that blow across the ocean towards land). They break for longer and in a gentle fashion when compared to other waves. They are the safest types of waves to swim in.

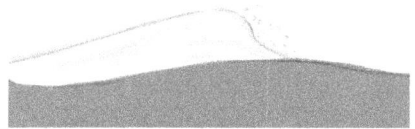

Plunging Waves

Plunging waves occur when the beach slope is moderate to steep or if it has a sudden change in depth, (a reef or sandbar, for example). They usually occur with offshore winds (winds that blow across the land towards the ocean) and at low tide.

These waves become more vertical than spilling waves and break with much more force. Experienced surfers often enjoy them for the tube they may create, but plunging waves have a lot more potential to cause serious injury to the swimmer. It's best to not swim in them.

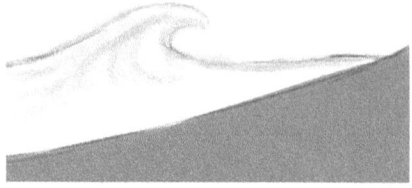

If caught in a plunging wave, hug your knees and roll up into a ball.

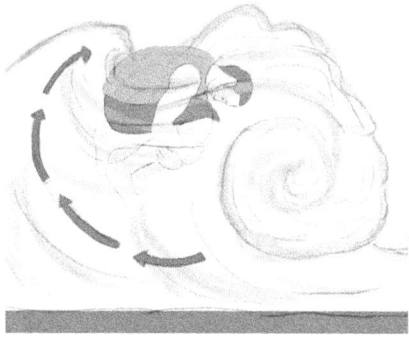

Surging Waves

Surging waves occur when long swells meet steep beach slopes. The bottom of these waves are fast enough that crests never form. As a result, there is little sign of breaking/whitewash.

Surging waves are dangerous. Although the wave break is minimal, the force of the waves is still powerful. They can knock you over and then drag you out to sea. Do not to swim when there are surging waves.

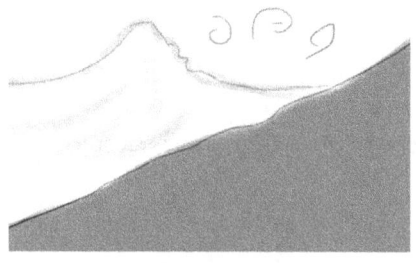

Another thing to be aware of is rough or choppy water. While it's not the same as a wave, it can still be hazardous. Rough seas can quickly drain your energy. It is best to get out and wait until the water is calm again.

Riding Waves to Shore

When the waves aren't too large you can use them to carry you to shore. Choose your wave and swim forward with it. Before it breaks, dive down a little so the break goes over you.

Large Waves

With larger surf, it is better to swim towards shore between oncoming waves. As a wave approaches, face it and go underwater until it has passed over you. Swim as far towards the shore as you can before repeating the process with the next wave. You may get caught in the undertow of a large wave. Get to the surface to avoid getting dragged out too far.

Rocky Shores

Only try to land on rocky shores if there is no other option. It's better to do a long-distance swim to an easier landing point than it is to risk injury on rocky shores. When you have to land on a rocky shore you must choose a safe landing point. Avoid ones where the waves crash into the rocks with a high white spray. Instead, aim for a spot where the waves rush up onto rocks. Once you know where you want to land, approach slowly. Use a large wave to carry you in. Get into the defensive position so you can absorb the impact.

If you do not reach the shore on the first wave, swim in the aggressive position with your hands only. When the next wave approaches, re-adopt the defensive position. When you climb up the rocks, keep your knees a little bent and your feet close together.

TIDES AND CURRENTS

Tides

The tide the rising and falling of the sea. High tide is when the water is at its highest level, and low tide is when it is at its lowest level. A few different natural forces influence tidal characteristics. It is important to check the tidal times depending on where and when you plan to visit the beach.

The change in water level due to tides can completely change the landscape within a short period of time. For example, if you walk out to a land mass in the morning, in the afternoon the path that you used may be underwater.

Currents

A current is a constant flow of water. It is always there, and it acts differently depending on water volume, channel width, gradient, weather, obstructions, etc.

Although you can use water currents in your favor, they can also take you where you do not want to go. Even slow ones can knock a person off his feet and carry him out to sea or downstream. Currents are usually slower along the inside bend of rivers than the outside bend, and are faster on the surface of the water.

Rip Currents

Rip currents can occur near beaches with breaking waves. They are strong currents that drag swimmers out to sea. Generally, the larger the waves, the stronger a rip current will be. The following characteristics can indicate a rip current:

- A channel of water that ripples more than the ones surrounding it.
- Dark water (indicates greater depth).
- Debris and/or sea-foam moving in a steady line out to sea.
- Different-colored water beyond the breaking waves.
- Murky water (indicates sand disturbed by the rip).
- Waves breaking further out to sea on both sides of the rip.

Look for a channel of water that is different (calmer or choppier) than the water surrounding it. A rip current may also be present with none of these characteristics showing.

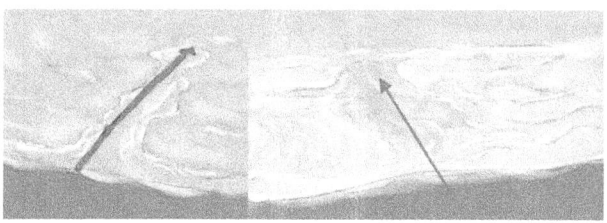

To escape a rip current:

- Do not try to swim against it!
- Stay calm.
- Swim parallel to the shore until you reach the breaking waves zone, then swim back to shore.
- If you can't escape it, conserve your energy (float or tread water) and signal for help.

In this picture, the thin arrows show the direction of the current. The four thicker arrows are your escape channels.

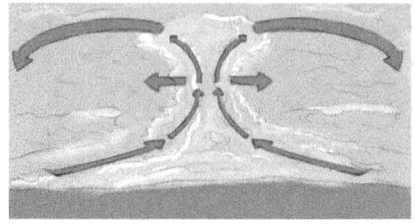

Related Chapters:

- Waves
- Obstructions

OBSTRUCTIONS

An obstruction is anything in the water that changes the normal current of the water. Almost anything in the water will do this, such as rocks, branches, etc. There are specific techniques to use depending on the obstruction you come across.

Drops

A drop is when water drops straight down. A waterfall is an obvious example. Never go in the water upstream from a drop. Even if the water is shallow and appears calm before the drop, it's still very dangerous. When going over a drop is unavoidable, ball up and try to land feet first. Landing feet first is the best way to protect your head. Balling up will lessen the possibility of getting caught in a foot entrapment. If it's a high drop, adopt the high-level entry position as you go over the edge.

Eddies

Eddies occur when water rushes around obstacles and the current comes back on itself. They are often safe havens, since the water in them is generally calmer. The point of separation between the upstream and downstream water is the eddy line. Problems can occur when you're crossing this line, especially if the flow is fast, but unless you're in a craft that can capsize, like a kayak, you shouldn't face much danger.

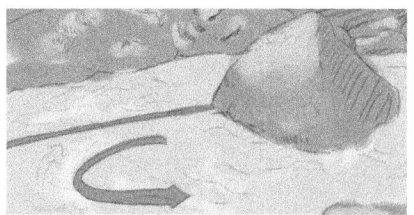

You can break through the eddy line with barrel rolls. As you approach the eddy, place your closest hand into the upstream-flowing water inside it. Scoop the water with this hand as you roll over onto your stomach. You are now in the aggressive swimming position. Continue to roll until you're back in the defensive swimming position.

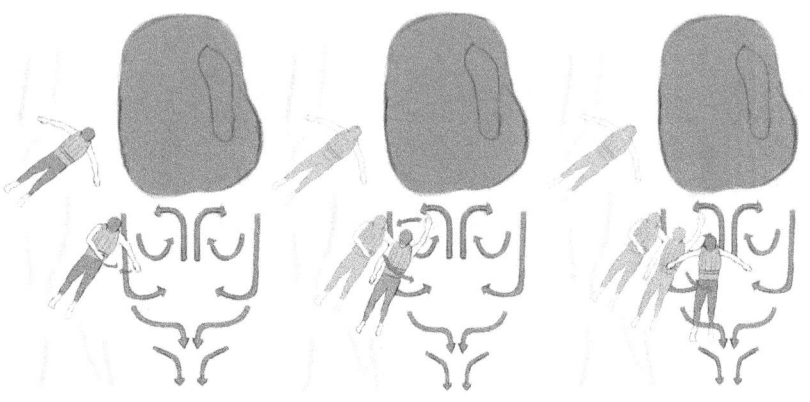

You may need to barrel roll a few times to get into the eddy. You can finish in either the defensive or aggressive swimming position. This image is a demonstration of using defensive and aggressive swimming to get out of a river.

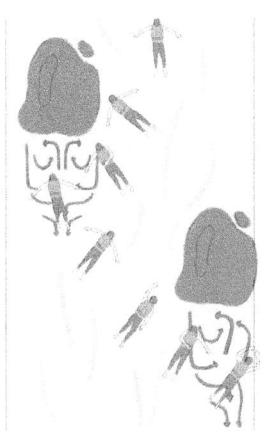

Sometimes an eddy can create a whirlpool effect. This is when eddies become dangerous, since the whirlpool can suck you down. In this case, you should stay clear of them.

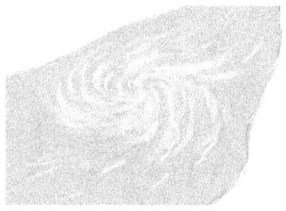

Entrapments

An entrapment is anything that you can get snagged on—an underwater branch that your clothing catches on, for example. To prevent this, make sure all your gear and clothing fits snugly.

A foot entrapment is when you get your foot stuck. It is very dangerous, as the force of the water can hold you under.

Holes

Holes occur when water flows over a ledge, such as a rock. This creates a hydraulic flow (water circulating on top of itself), which can trap things. It's like a vertical eddy, and is very dangerous.

Dams and dam-like structures (weirs, spillways, ledges) have severe hydraulic action. Keep away from their downstream bases.

If you're caught in a hole, you need to relax and swim out the bottom (where the slower current flows out) or to the side.

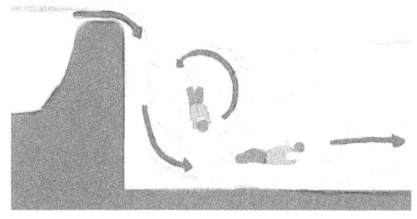

Pillows

When a rock is close to the water's surface, the water hits the top of it, forcing it upwards. This creates a "pillow" of water downstream from the rock.

The more submerged a rock is, the further downstream the pillow will be. If the rock is very close to the surface, the pillow will be right on top of it. With enough experience, you will be able to tell when a rock is close to the surface or not by the type of pillow it creates.

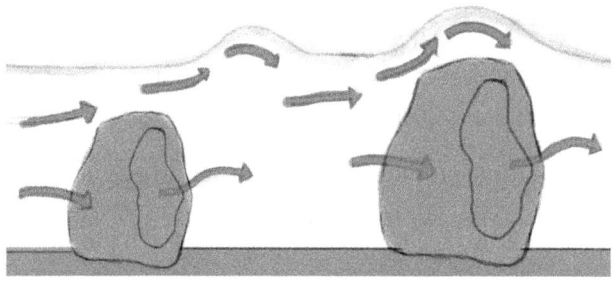

If the rock is out of the water, the pillow becomes a cushion. This is due to the water flowing up against it. When the current is strong enough, it may form a series of compression waves.

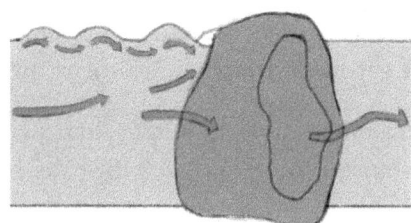

Rapids

A rapid is a turbulent section of water created by water flowing faster over obstacles, such as rocks. These obstacles may or may not break the water's surface. This faster water is due to an increased gradient and/or a constriction in the channel.

To negotiate a rapid, look for a downstream "V" in the water (the bottom of the V will point downstream). This indicates an unobstructed flow of water. In most cases, it will be the preferred passage.

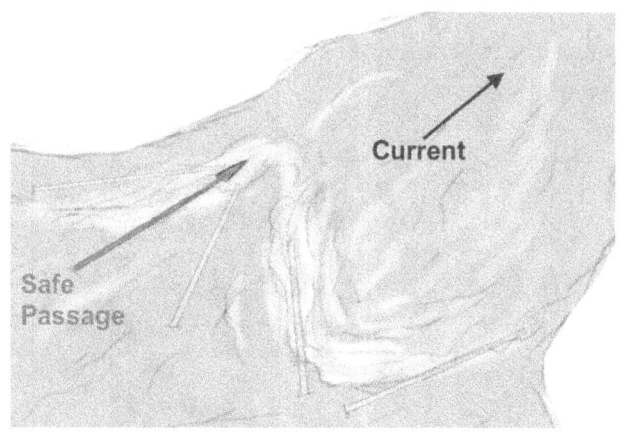

Rocks

Apart from being a cause for other types of obstructions, a rock itself can present danger. Avoid these obstructions altogether by entering the water downstream from them.

Walking on slippery rocks (or any slippery surface) near water is never a good idea.

Rocks under the water's surface can become foot entrapments. They're very dangerous and are one of the main reasons to keep your feet up in the defensive position.

When you're in the water heading towards a rock, use the defensive position, as described before. If you get pinned up against one, lean downstream to get loose.

Rocks are not all bad. They may serve as lifelines to hold onto. They can also create eddies, which can be safe havens in turbulent waters.

Sweepers and Strainers

Strainers are objects in the water that allow water to pass through them, but not other objects. They can be natural, like branches, or artificial, like wire fences.

A sweeper is a strainer that hangs low over or into the water.

Both of these things can impede your safe passage, and they often double as entrapments.

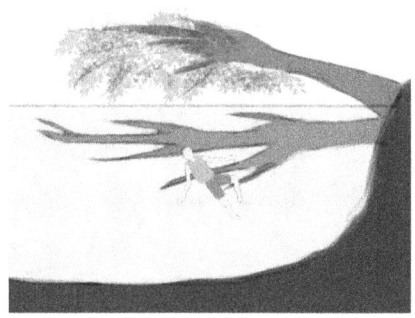

When swimming into a strainer is unavoidable, maneuver into the aggressive swimming position. Swim hard to launch yourself up and onto (or over) the obstruction.

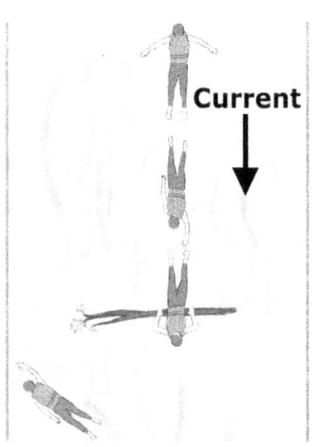

When forced below the surface, swim downstream, with your hands in front of you to part the branches. If your legs get tangled in long weeds, swim downstream using only your arms.

Like friendly rocks, sometimes sweepers (though not strainers) can serve as lifelines. You might be able to use them to climb to shore.

Undercut Rocks

An undercut rock is one the water flows below, as opposed to around. The water's current can drag a swimmer underneath it and pin him there.

Normal river features acting strangely are good indications of an undercut rock. For example, you might see that:

- The pillow or cushion is missing.
- There is a boil (where the water is not flowing down or upstream) on the downstream side of the obstacle.
- The eddy has weak or missing lines, and/or an abnormal current flow.

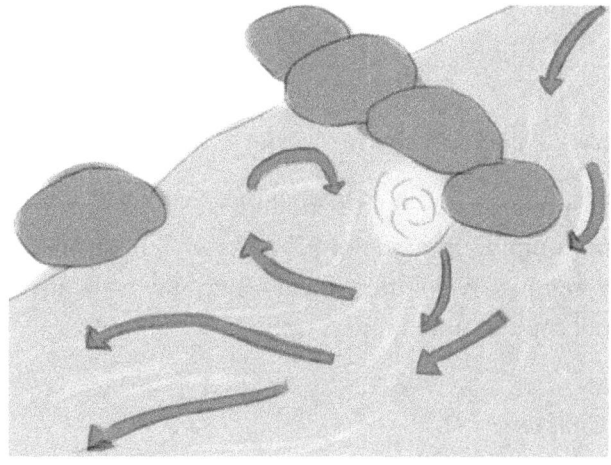

Water Debris

Water debris is anything floating in the water. It can be either natural or unnatural, such as seaweed, logs, trash, etc. Keep an eye out for these things and avoid them, as they can become entrapments.

If there is a lot of debris, such as lots of seaweed, try to avoid it. If you must go through it, crawl over the top of it by grasping at it with over-hand movements. When you are in a group, put the strongest person first. He will create a path through the debris for the others to follow.

Manmade pools created behind dams often have many stumps lying below the surface. This is due to the cutting of trees before the flooding of the lowlands.

People

Other people can be a hazard, although they are more often a good thing in a survival situation.

There are more recreational hazards, like surfers, jet-skis, and boats, in open water. Stay away from areas in which these activities take place. Use the designated swimming areas instead, if those are available.

Pollution

Another byproduct of people is pollution. Water systems are often used as a dumping ground for all sorts of human and industrial waste. Swimming in polluted waters may not have an immediate effect, but it could result in illness later.

Related Chapters:

- Waves

SELF-RESCUE BOWLINE

The self-rescue bowline is good to learn in case you find yourself in a "man overboard" situation or something similar. It's a bowline tied around your waist with only one hand. To make one:

Wrap the rope around your waist so that both the standing and running ends are to your front with your body (waist) between them. In this demonstration, the running end is on your right.

Hold the running end in your right hand allowing at least 15cm of rope beyond your hand. Without letting go of the running end, bring it over the standing part to make a crossing point. Bring it up though the gap created between your body and the crossing point. The rope will be wrapped around your hand.

Using your fingers, but without letting go of the rope, pass the running end under the standing part just beyond the first crossing point. This creates a second crossing point.

Continue to maneuver the running end with your fingers so that it feeds between the two crossing points. It feeds from the top down. It should end with you holding the running end.

Once that is accomplished, pull your hand out from the loop on your wrist, bringing the running end with you. Pull the knot tight.

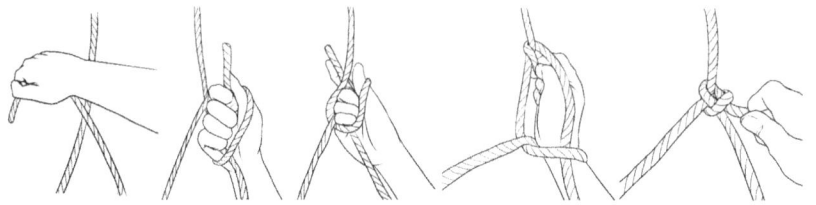

IMPROVISED FLOTATION AIDS

Any medium-sized object that floats—a football, Styrofoam cooler, floating log, etc.—can aid you when you're swimming across a body of water. Tying together smaller empty containers also works well in slow water.

Tie your flotation device to your wrist and grab onto it if you get tired.

You could also hug it with one arm, although you would need to improvise your stroke. Sidestroke would work well for this.

Inflating Your Clothes

Being stranded in the water and having to tread water to stay afloat expends precious energy.

When you are wearing long pants or a long-sleeved shirt, you can trap air inside them to help you float.

These methods work best with waterproof materials. If you have cotton clothing, keep the material that is out of the water wet to prevent air escaping.

Inflating Your Top

As you tread water (feet only), pull up your collar and bunch your shirt around your mouth to make a tight seal. Keep your nose out in the open. Breathe in through your nose and exhale out your mouth into your shirt. Direct air into your shoulder area by leaning forward.

Inflating Your Pants

If you can't take your pants off over your shoes, remove the shoes. Tie the laces together, and then hang them around your neck.

Remove your pants, do the zipper up, and tie the bottoms of the legs together. Inflate the legs using the blow, sling, or splash method.

After inflating your pants, keep the waistband underwater. Put your head between the legs and hug the pants, with the fly facing your body. Fold or twist the waistband closed to create a seal.

You can rest your head back on the knot. Keep the exposed material wet by splashing water on it. If you need to, open the waistband (while keeping it underwater) and scoop more air in.

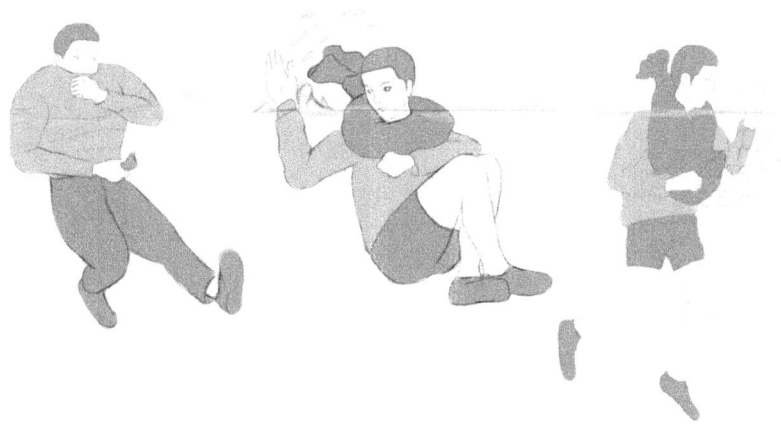

Blow Method

This method is best for weak swimmers.

Hold your pants the right way up by the waistband, with the fly facing you. Take a deep breath and go underwater with the pants.

Blow air into them. Keeping the pants underwater, take another breath and blow more air into them. Repeat this until they are filled with air.

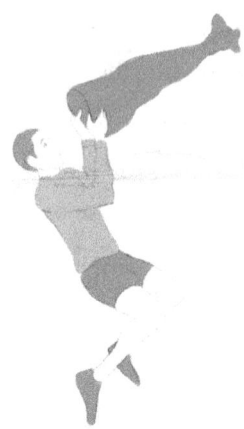

Sling Method

Hold the pants behind your head by the waistband, ensuring you keep it open. Using a forceful motion, sling the pants over your head in front of you and into the water to fill them with air.

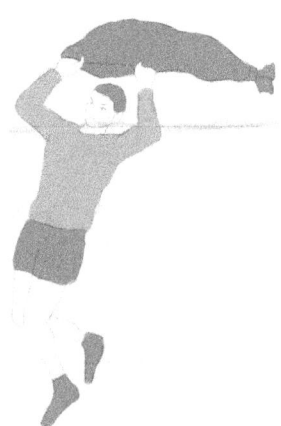

Splash Method

Hold the waistband open underwater with one hand, fly facing up and pants on the surface. With your other hand inside the waistband, scoop water and air bubbles into your pants. Scoop quickly. The water will pass through, leaving the air trapped.

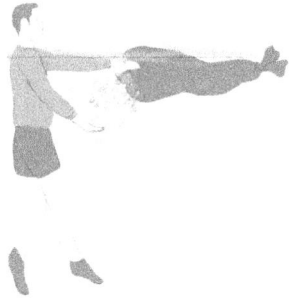

Related Chapters:

- Swimming Across

COLD WATER SURVIVAL

Being immersed in cold water will sap your breath and energy quicker than normal. Panicking will make things worse. You must relax and get out. Concentrate on deep breathing to calm your mind and body.

If you cannot get onto dry land, you have to do whatever you can to conserve your body heat until help arrives. Take these steps:

- Button or zip up your clothes and keep them on.
- Don't use up energy swimming unless you have a dry place to swim to.
- Get as much of yourself out of the water as possible.
- Use the H.E.L.P. or huddle position.

Once you get out of the water, it's important to remove all your wet clothing, dry yourself off, and get warm. Watch yourself and others for signs of hypothermia, and treat them as needed. There is more information about hypothermia and other cold-related illnesses in the bonus section.

H.E.L.P

H.E.L.P. is an acronym for the Heat Escape Lessening Posture. It's the position to adopt when you're alone in the water and want to conserve your body heat. The general idea of H.E.L.P. is to protect your major heat-loss areas—that is, your armpits, groin, head, neck, and ribcage.

When you're wearing a life-jacket, keep your head out of the water and lean back on it. Fold your arms and hug your jacket close to your body. Cross your lower legs and bring your knees as high on your chest as you can.

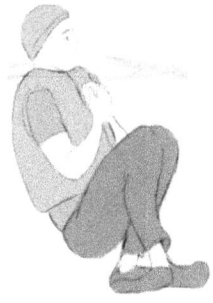

If you don't have a life jacket, do your best to get as close to H.E.L.P. as possible.

Huddle Position

The huddle position is H.E.L.P. for groups of two or more people. Huddling together in a group has benefits such as:

- Lessening the loss of body heat.
- Increasing morale.
- Be easier for rescuers to spot.
- Allowing stronger swimmers to aid weaker ones.

To adopt the huddle position, form a ring and group together as closely as possible. Wrap your arms and legs around each other. Place those who are vulnerable (such as children) in the middle.

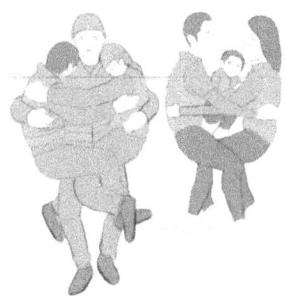

Falling Through Ice

Escaping from a fall into ice water is not easy, and the result can be deadly.

DO NOT PRACTICE THIS IN ICE WATER! Go through the motions in a pool instead.

When you first fall into ice water, you'll start to hyperventilate. Try to stay calm and keep your head above the water. Taking deep breaths may help, but be careful not to breathe in any of the water.

After one to three minutes, the shock response will begin to wear off. Now you'll have about 10 minutes to get out before you fall unconscious. Once you have your hyperventilation under control, find where you first fell in. You want to get out where you know the ice was strong enough to support your weight, so going back to where you came from is your best bet.

Place your hands on the surface and pull yourself up, while staying as flat to the ice as possible. Pulling yourself straight up will be far less effective and a waste of energy.

Kick your legs as you creep out of the water. It will be very slippery.

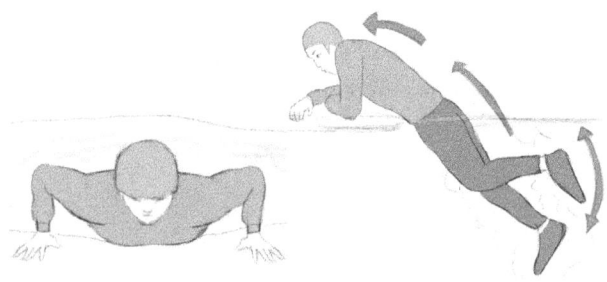

Once you are out of the water, lie flat on the ice and roll away. Rolling keeps your weight distributed, and has less of a chance of creating further cracks in the ice. Get out of your wet clothes and get warm as soon as possible.

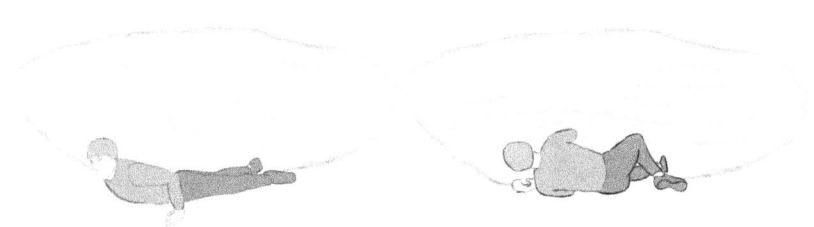

If you know you'll be crossing ice country, it's very wise to get some ice picks. They will make it far easier to pull yourself out of the water, although it will still be difficult.

At the very least, put some large nails in your pocket to help you grip the ice when you need to pull yourself out.

If you can't get out, you need to conserve your heat and energy. Put your arms on the ice and keep them there, so that they freeze to the surface. That way, when you lose consciousness, you'll have a better chance of not falling into the water.

Never go out to someone who has fallen into ice. Coach them on what to do from a safe distance, and hold something out for them to grab onto, such as a stick or a rope.

FLOOD

A flood occurs when water covers land that is normally dry. Common causes are heavy rain, snow melt, and massive ocean waves.

Minor flooding is usually not a problem, but large floods can be quite destructive. The higher up you are, the safer you'll be from flooding.

When you're caught in a flood, get inside a building. Prepare your survival kits and some kind of raft. Even a floating door is better than nothing. Turn off the gas, electricity, and water at the mains, then move to an upper floor or roof with a shelter. If the building has a sloping roof, tie everyone on. Unless you live on the coast or are forced to evacuate, stay put.

Evacuating

To evacuate in a flood, seek shelter on the highest ground possible.

Do not attempt to cross water unless you're certain that it won't be higher than the center of your vehicle's wheels, or your knees if you're on foot. Even a small drop can make a big difference in water level. Be careful of a bridge already underwater. It may be missing.

If your car dies, abandon it.

After the Flood

Contamination of food and water is high after a flood, so stay away from floodwater and fresh food that has come into contact with floodwater.

You can eat canned food that has been exposed to floodwater. Wash the cans with soap and clean, hot water before opening them. Purify all water before consuming it.

SWIMMING WHEN RESTRAINED

When you're restrained and thrown in the water, use the CSS kick (Swimming Long Distance) to propel you forward. If your captors also restrain your legs, use the dolphin kick.

The challenging part is getting your head above the water to take a breath.

Bring your knees to your stomach.

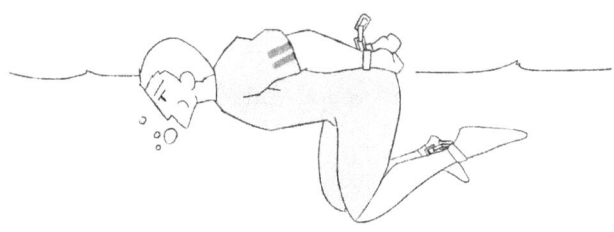

Kick both back at once as you arch your back to propel your head out of the water.

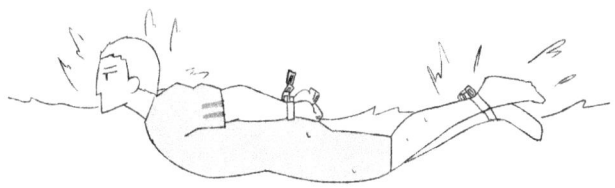

Take a breath, and then return to the dolphin kick until you need to do it again.

In rough waters, rotate your body so you are on your back to take a breath. This prevents you accidentally inhaling water.

SURVIVAL AT SEA

Sea survival is tough. Use the information in this chapter to give you the best chance of staying alive and getting rescued.

Abandoning Ship

When you suspect you may need to abandon ship, or if your plane will crash in the ocean, put on warm (preferably woolen) clothing. Cover as much of your body as you can and put on a life jacket. Gather whatever survival provisions you can, and get to a lifeboat. Do not exceed the maximum capacity of a life vessel. Have the healthy hang off the side and swap regularly.

If you have to jump from the ship:

- Throw something that floats in first, and jump to it.
- Wait until you are off the ship before inflating your life jacket.
- Once you're in the sea, get upwind and away from the sinking vessel.

When you don't have a flotation device, grab whatever you might be able to use to build a raft or attract the attention of a rescue craft using noise and light.

Failing that, keep composed and swim steadily upwind of the sinking vessel. If there is a chance of an underwater explosion, swim on your back. Swim under any danger such as fire.

Life Rafts

When you have an inflatable life raft, wait until you're clear of the wreck before inflating it, unless you can board it and stay dry.

Inflate the raft to the point it's firm, but not too hard. Compensate for the surrounding temperature (heat makes air expand). Do not jump into it, and make sure nothing can puncture it. Secure all passengers and equipment to it. Waterproof everything that requires it. Check for leaks and the inflation level at least once daily. If you see little bubbles, it's a sign of leaks. Repair them ASAP.

To board a life raft from the water, move to one end (not the side). Put one leg over the edge and roll inside. If the life raft has a line attached, grab the line on the opposite side from where it is attached. Brace your feet against the raft and pull yourself in. Expect the other end of the life raft to come up. You can improvise this to right an overturned life raft.

To help someone else on board, hold him by his shoulders and get him to lift one leg over the end of the raft (if possible). Roll him in.

Survival at Sea

If rescue is likely and there is no land in sight, or if you're near regular shipping lanes, wait close to the crash site for rescue for at least 72 hours. If you see land or know that it's near, head for it.

Assign lookouts on short shifts. Look for signs of life, land, rescue, leaks, and anything that could be useful. Keep your position by making a sea anchor. Tie weighted objects to a line.

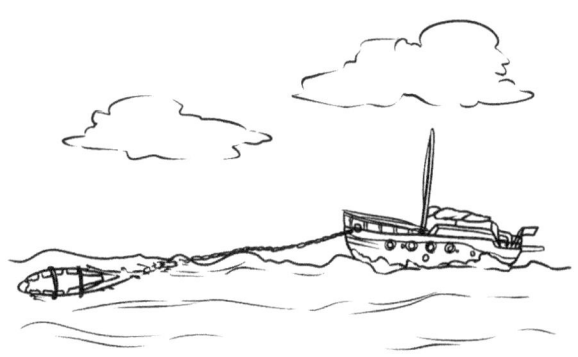

Ration water and food immediately, even if you expect rescue. Use whistles and lights to maintain contact with others if visibility is poor.

Movement at Sea

When you're lost at sea, your main aim is to find rescue or land. To do that, you need to use either the current or the wind to take you to where you want to go.

To use the current, deflate your raft a little so it rides low in the water. Deploy your sea anchor and keep low in the raft.

To use the wind, you need a sail. Inflate the raft so it rides higher, pull the sea anchor in, and sit up so your body catches the wind.

If you improvise a sail, prevent the raft from capsizing by holding the bottom with your hands, so you can release it quickly if there is a sudden gust of wind.

When in rough waters, keep low and stream the sea anchor from the bow (front). Tying life vessels together will improve their stability.

Landing

In most cases, surviving on land is much easier than surviving at sea. Look for the following signs of land:

- A constant wind with a decreasing swell. Land is windward.
- A green tint on the undersides of clouds.
- Isolated cumulus clouds.
- Muddy water, indicating silt from a large river mouth.
- Lighter-colored water, indicating shallow water.
- Seabirds flying. They move away from land before noon and return to it in the afternoon.
- Odors and sounds of land, including smoke, vegetation, surf, animals, etc.

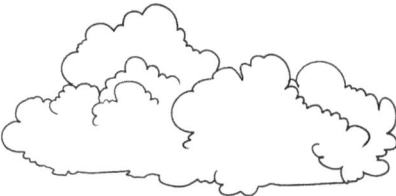

Cumulus clouds are "puffy" with flat bases.

Once you find land, you need to get to it safely. Wait until daytime to choose a landing point, and select one from which it will be easy to beach or swim ashore. The downwind side of an island is usually better.

As you approach the shore, assess the features of the landscape (high ground, vegetation, water courses, etc.). Choose a meeting point in case you get separated. Secure all your gear to your body and have a flotation aid ready. Stay in the raft for as long as possible.

Take down the sail and put a sea anchor out to keep you pointing at the shore, unless you're going through coral. Head for gaps in the surf. Waves usually occur in sets of seven, from small to large. Steer clear of rocks, ice, and other obstacles.

When you get close, paddle hard and use the waves to carry you into shore. If the surf is heavy, point towards the sea and paddle into approaching waves. To avoid getting swept back out to sea, make the raft as light as possible and take out the sea anchor.

When the undercurrent tries to take you back out, fill part of the raft with water and stream the anchor towards the shore.

Swimming to Shore

To swim to shore, face it and sit with your feet about a meter below your head so you can take any impact on the bottoms of your feet. If the surf is high, swim towards the shore in the trough between waves.

When a wave going out to sea approaches, go under it, then continue to the shore. For more information, see the Tides and Currents chapter.

Related Chapters:

- Waves
- Tides and Currents

RIVER CROSSINGS

When crossing a body of water with no bridge, you need to use river-crossing techniques. They will give you the best chance of making it to the other side unharmed.

CHOOSING WHERE TO CROSS

It is very important to find a safe crossing point before attempting to cross. When practical (and not dangerous), it is best to scout the river from an elevated perspective.

Unless you can jump it, narrow is not best. Look for straight, wide, and shallow water. The current is faster at the bends and usually deeper in narrow channels. Lots of debris is also a sign of fast flow. Test the current by throwing a branch in and seeing how fast it goes. Mild ripples are generally safe to cross. Whitecaps (small, surface-breaking waves) will be slippery.

Although it may be wider, the point where a river breaks into channels is usually a good crossing location. The energy of the current dissipates there, and there may be small patches of land where you can take breaks. Check 100m (33ft) downstream of where you plan to cross. Make sure there aren't any hazards you could be swept into. Consider your entry and exit points. An easy exit point is especially important. You want something low and open so you don't have to climb through or up anything.

You may be able to avoid getting wet if you find a fallen log that spans the width of the river.

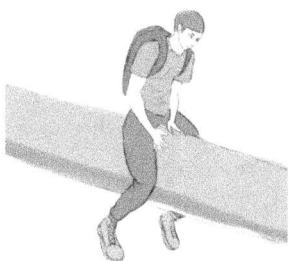

If you do find one, don't try to walk over it. It is much safer to straddle it and scoot yourself across. You must be very sure it will hold your weight. When you're in a group, have only one person cross at a time.

WATERPROOFING YOUR PACK

A waterproofed pack will not only keep all your kit dry, it can also be an effective flotation device.

Double waterproof everything at the very least.

Line your pack with a large, tough, plastic bag. If you don't want to buy a pack liner, then you can use a dead-dog bag from the vet. Even a large, tough, plastic trash bag will work.

Group your things into separate, smaller dry-sacks before putting them in your pack. You could use plastic bags and/or zip-locks.

Seal all the bags watertight by following the manufacturer's directions.

For generic plastic bags use the twist and fold method. Leave enough space at the top so you can put several twists in the bag. Fold the twisted part down over itself and secure it with some twine.

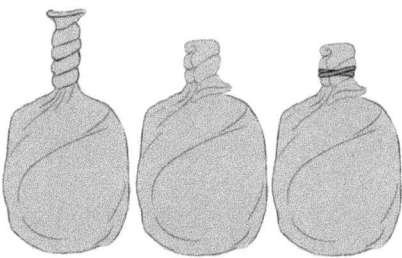

It may be faster to line your pack with two large bags but using this method works better. It means you can access one group of things without having to expose everything else to the elements.

WADING

Wading is a method of walking through water. Use it in water no deeper than thigh height. When wading, you can take your pants, shirt, and socks off to lessen the water's drag. Doing this will also give you dry clothes on the other side.

Keep your shoes on. You won't want to risk damaging your feet, and you will want the traction shoes will provide.

Tie your clothing to the top of your pack, or in one bundle if you don't have a pack. The idea is to keep everything together so it's easier to find if you have to discard it while crossing.

If you're wading across with a pack, carry it on your shoulders. Leave your waist belt unclipped and loosen your shoulder straps, so you can discard the pack if necessary. You won't want to be struggling to get it off if the current sweeps you off your feet. Don't worry about having a heavy pack when crossing. It will keep you more stable.

Solo Wading

If you're wading alone, use a strong branch to support you as you cross. Three legs are far more stable than two.

Position yourself upstream of your chosen exit point so that you can cross at a 45-degree angle to the current. Face upstream and place the tip of your branch on the bottom of the river in front of you. Keep it slanted and let the current push it against your shoulder. Your branch will break the current and provide stability. Shuffle sideways and a little downstream across the river. Use small, low steps. Do not cross your feet.

Always maintain at least two points of contact with the bottom of the river. Don't move too far on either side of your branch. You don't want to be leaning.

Only reposition the branch once your feet are very stable on the river floor. Shift it in small increments, feeling for your next placement. Lift it off the river floor only as much as you need to.

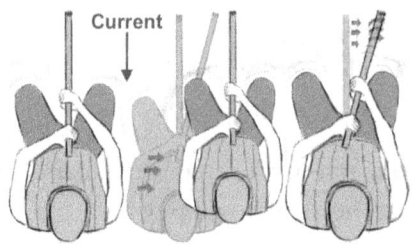

Group Wading

When two or more people need to get across, you can use group wading.

The technique differs a little depending on how many people you have.

If two people wading, the stronger person should be upstream, and facing downstream. The second person should face the first person (looking upstream).

Grab each other by the shoulder straps of each other's life jackets. If you don't have lifejackets, grab t-shirts or upper arms.

One person stays stationary while the other moves. Use the same small sideways steps as explained above. Next, the other moves and the first person stays still. Repeat this process as needed.

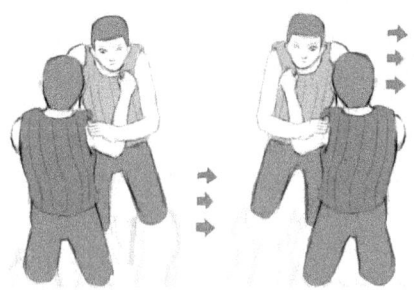

Groups of three to five people should huddle together, with each person grabbing the people on either side of him. One or more people stay stationary while the rest move. Due to the group formation, you may end up rotating the group around the stationary person/people. It is okay to do this.

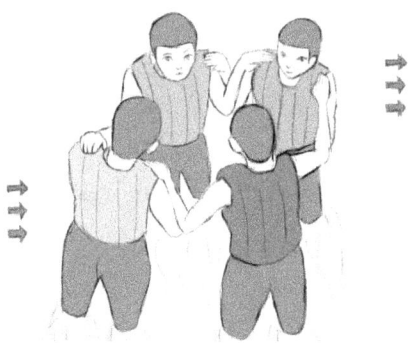

Wading in groups larger than five is not recommended, as it becomes too hard to coordinate.

As with all group coordination activities, clear communication is very important. Agree on a plan of movement beforehand and appoint one person to direct it as you go.

Inline Crossing

Use inline crossing to move larger numbers of inexperienced people. With this method, you use your bodies to redirect the current so people can move behind each other.

The strongest person enters the water first, facing upstream. The second person moves behind the first, and takes up his position immediately to the side of that person. They link arms.

Everyone else copies this action until they form one line across the water. More than one person can move at a time.

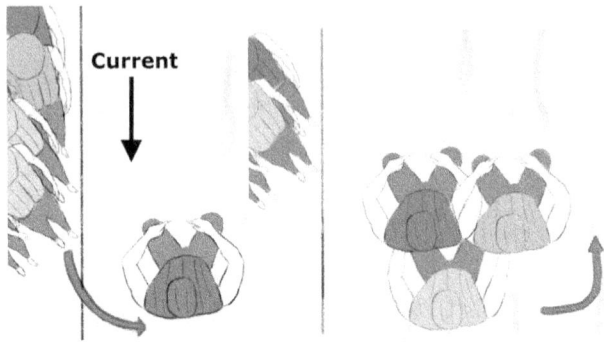

Once the line is steady, the first person moves down it to take his new position at the end.

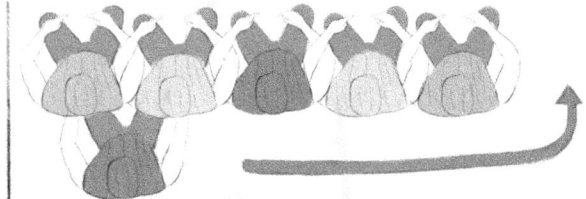

Everyone does this in the order that they entered, repeating the action until the line reaches the other side and everyone is on shore.

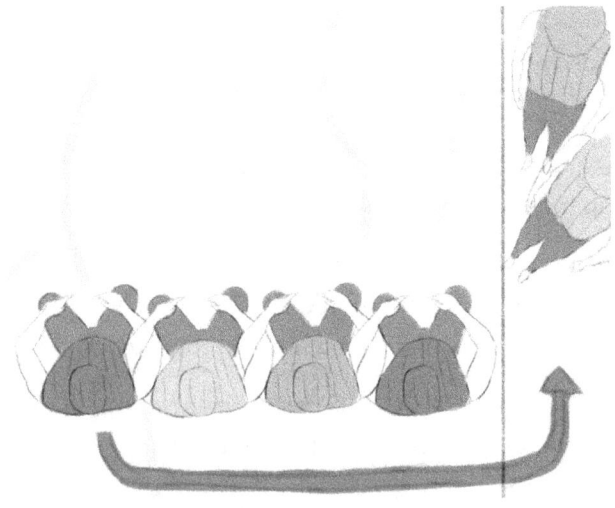

ROPE CROSSINGS

Having a rope increases your safety when you're crossing water, and may also increase your speed. This chapter assumes you only have rope, and no other specialist equipment.

Looped Rope Crossing

This is one of the safest ways to cross a river when you have a rope but no other special equipment. You need at least three people and a rope three times the width of the river.

The first and last people to cross should be the strongest in the group, with the stronger of the two going first.

Tie the rope into a large loop and secure the person who is going to cross first (person A) in the loop by putting it over his chest. As person A crosses, the other two people let the rope out as needed. They must do their best to keep the rope out of the water and be ready to haul person A back if needed.

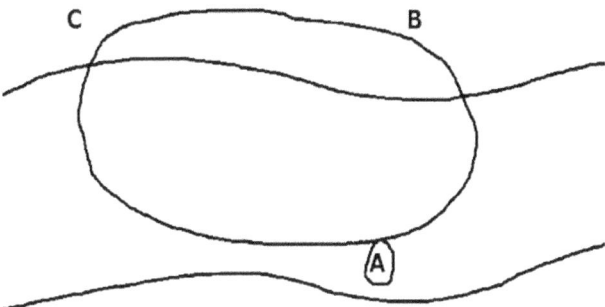

Person A is the only one secured to the rope.

When person A reaches the other side, he unties himself.

As many people as needed can now cross (B), one at a time, by securing themselves to the rope and crossing over.

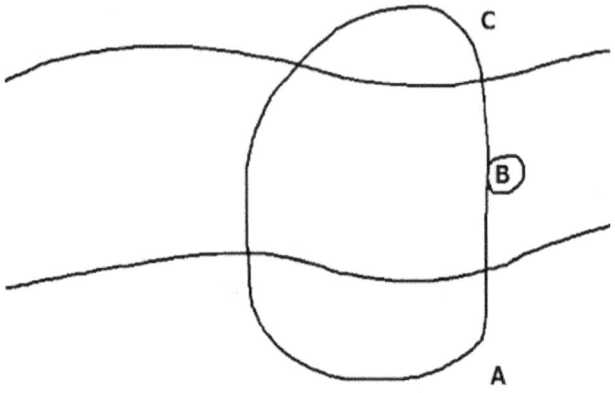

Extra people can help while others are crossing, but person A takes most of the strain. This person should be as close as possible to the position across from the person crossing.

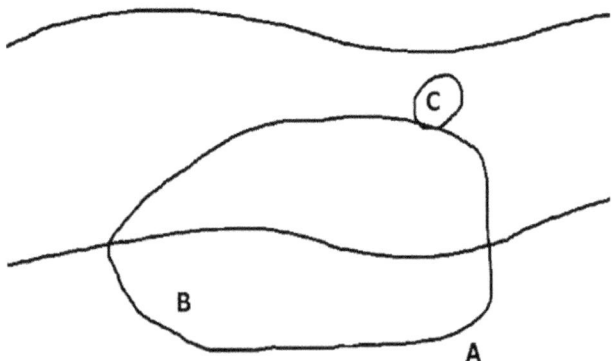

Line Crossing

When you don't have enough rope and/or people to do the looped rope crossing, you can use a line crossing.

Stretch the rope across the water and secure it on both ends. To do this, you must get one end of the rope across the other side of the river.

If there is already someone on the other side, you can throw it over. If not, you can attach one end of the rope to the strongest swimmer (or wader) in the group and have him take it over.

It is preferable not to attach the rope directly to the swimmer. If possible, attach it to the back of his life jacket instead. That way, it will be easier for him to discard the line if needed.

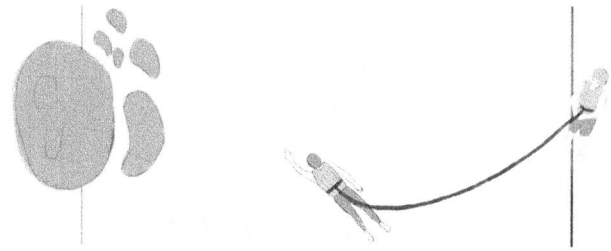

If you must attach the rope directly to the swimmer, you can use a bowline.

One person should feed the line out as the swimmer crosses. When feeding the line out, let it drift in the current to reduce drag on the swimmer.

Note: *There is more information on swimming across in the Swimming Across chapter.*

To secure the rope, tie it to a sturdy tree, rock, or something similar. If nothing else is available, you can use a human anchor. When doing so, it's best to have at least one other person pushing down on him so he doesn't get dragged into the water.

Once the rope is secure on both sides, people can start wading across. Wade across facing the current, using the rope for support. Apply tension to the line by leaning back a little. This will help keep you stable. Do not cross your legs as you wade across, and only move one foot at a time.

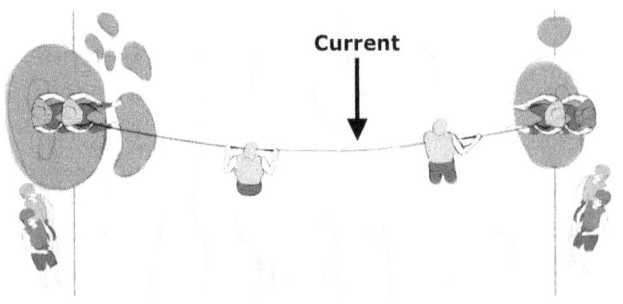

To keep the rope, the last person must release the knot and then attach himself to it. The people on the other side can pull him across if needed.

Throwing Rope

Knowing the correct way to throw rope will increase the distance you can throw it. In most cases, you should aim to over-throw it. If you intend to keep one end of the rope (which is usually the case), be sure to secure it to something.

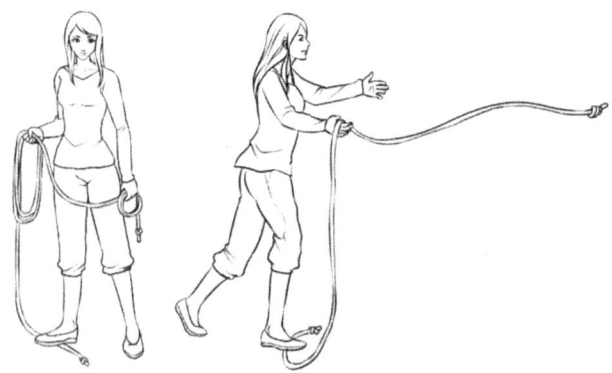

Even when you're throwing all the rope to someone, it's a good idea to secure one end. If your throw doesn't clear the obstacle, you can pull it back. If it does, then untie your end and let the other person pull it over.

Tie a weight or a bulky stopper knot to the end you're going to throw over. Coil half the rope on the palm of your right hand, and the rest of it on your fingers. Stand on one end to secure it, or tie it to something.

Grab the coils you made on your fingers with your left hand. As you throw, release the right-hand coil a split second before the left.

When throwing a weighted rope over a branch, beware of it swinging back.

Related Chapters:

- Wading
- Swimming Across

BUILDING AN IMPROVISED RAFT

If the water body you want to cross is too wide, deep, cold, and/or contains dangerous animals, it's a good idea to build a raft. This will also help keep you and your gear dry.

Building a raft can be very helpful, but if you do it wrong, the results can be disastrous.

Build the raft near the water body in which you want to launch it.

Improvised rafts are not suitable for the ocean. It's unlikely that they will stand up to the force of an angry sea.

There are many ways to build a raft. You can use bamboo, wood, or other floating objects.

Always test your raft before committing to using it.

Brush Raft

If you have a couple of ponchos, you can construct a brush raft. When done right, it can float over 100 kilograms, which is enough for one average-sized person and his kit.

A tarpaulin (groundsheet) or something similar also works, as long as it's waterproof and about the same size as a poncho.

Spread one poncho on the ground with the inner side facing the sky. Tie a length of cord (vines work) at each corner, and another in the center of each side. Each line must be long enough to reach the opposite diagonal or side. If there aren't dedicated tie points (grommets), then you can bunch up the material in a package around a small rock. Tie a clove hitch below the rock. The rock will prevent the knot from slipping off.

Pile fresh, green brush on top of the poncho, about half a meter high. It must be all brush, not thick branches or anything that could pierce the ponchos. Next, find two small saplings and construct an x-frame. Place this x-frame on top of the brush.

Pile another 50 cm of brush on top of that. Push down on it all to compress it a little. Pull the sides of the poncho up and around the brush, and then tie all the lines together with their opposites. Tie them very securely.

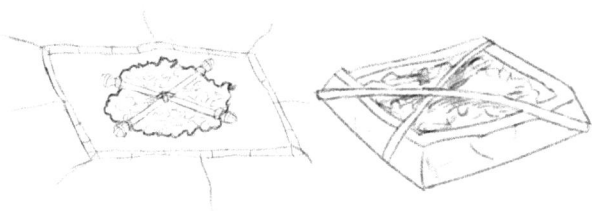

Spread the second poncho on the ground next to your brush package, with the inner side facing the sky. Tie cord at the corners and the sides in the same way as the first time. Place your brush package onto the second poncho, with the tied side facing down.

Secure it in the same manner. When you place the brush raft in the water, do it with the tied side of the second poncho facing up.

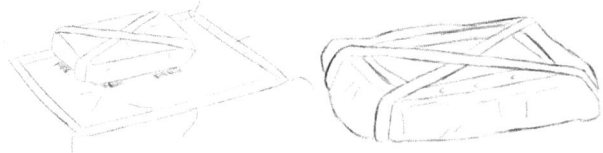

Pressure Raft

A pressure raft takes a lot more effort to build than a brush raft. The tradeoff is that it's much sturdier and can support much more weight.

It's best to use dry, dead, standing trees for logs, but remember that not all wood floats. Test the species you intend to use before constructing the raft.

Collect logs of approximately the same diameter and make them the same length. These are your base logs. How many base logs you collect depends on how wide you want the raft to be.

When you've collected your base logs, gather four thinner ones. These should be about one meter longer than the thickness of the raft. They are your pressure logs.

Lay two pressure logs on the ground at a distance from each other that's about one meter less than the length of the base logs. Lay the base logs on top of the pressure logs so that they are perpendicular to them. The ends should have enough overhang that they can't slip off.

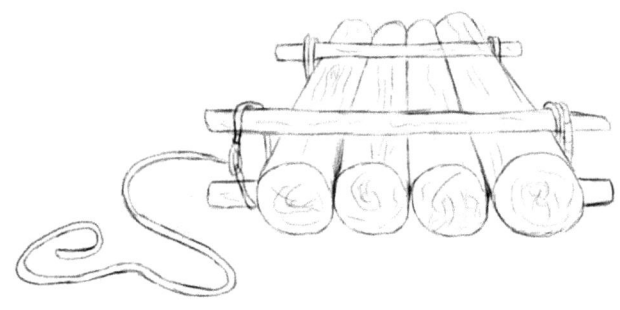

Place the other two pressure logs on top of the thicker ones. Align them, and ensure they're parallel to the pressure logs on the bottom.

Tie the ends of the top and bottom pressure logs together at all corners, so they clamp the raft together. Do so as tight as you can.

Bamboo Raft

Bamboo is one of the best materials for raft building. It is strong, flexible, and floats well.

Note: Bamboo that has not dried out can sink. It can take a while for it to dry out if it is freshly cut.

Cut relative thick bamboo in 3-meter lengths. If it's too hard to cut down, you can burn it at its base until it falls. Make holes in the lower sections before burning it to prevent it from exploding.

Make holes in each of the lengths about 30 cm from the ends and in the center. Make sure the holes will be in alignment when you put the lengths side by side.

Place the bamboo side by side until you get your desired width. Pass a sapling through all the holes. Create a second row in the same manner, using one less length of bamboo. Place this second row on top of the first, with the lengths of the top row sitting in the valleys of the first. Tie the lengths of bamboo together, top and bottom and side by side. Tie the saplings together as well.

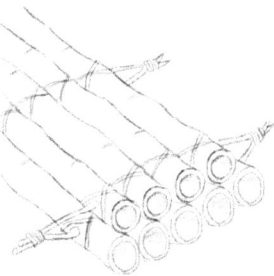

You can do this with materials other than bamboo too, but bamboo works best.

Tips for Traveling by Raft

Always test your raft before committing to taking it across a water body. Keep near the shore if possible, and head to the bank if the raft gets out of control.

If you're rafting between islands, do so when the ebb takes you out and the high tide takes you to the new island. Study the currents by floating something you can observe.

If there are several rafts full of people, put one carrying a scouting party out in front. It should hold the most capable members of the group and minimal equipment.

Use a pole to move the raft through shallow water, and an oar to move it through deep water.

Stay near the inside edges of river bends. The current will be slower there.

Tie all equipment to the raft and make sure nothing trails over the edges.

Tie everyone to the raft (use a bowline around the waist), except in swift water. Lifelines should allow free movement, but should not trail in the water.

Avoid obstructions.

When you come across rapids (or other dangerous ground) do the following:

- Unload the raft and secure it to the bank.
- Carry all equipment downstream by land.
- If the raft is too heavy to carry past the obstacle, place at least one member downstream from the raft. He should be at a safe spot where he'll be able to recover it.
- Release the raft.
- Be sure to make repairs if needed.

At night, secure the raft well, and take shelter on high ground, away from the river.

SWIMMING ACROSS

Swimming across a river is a last resort, but you may have to. When doing so, you must allow for the drag of the current. Choose your exit point, and then choose an entry point upstream. How far upstream you need to enter depends on the strength of the current and how strong of a swimmer you are. Use your best judgment.

Use the aggressive swimming technique (freestyle, with your head above water).

When there is more than one swimmer, it's a good idea to pair (or triple if there is an odd number) them up. Pair a good swimmer who knows proper rescue techniques with a weak one so he can help if needed.

Improvised Flotation Aids

Any medium-sized object that floats—a football, Styrofoam cooler, floating log, etc.—can aid you when you're swimming across a body of water. Tying together smaller, empty containers also works well in slow water.

Tie your flotation device to your wrist and grab onto it if you get tired. You could also hug it with one arm, although you would need to improvise your stroke. Sidestroke would work well for this.

Floating Pack

Waterproofing your pack as described before will give it some buoyancy.

If you know you'll need the pack as a flotation device, trap air inside the pack liner before sealing it off. It's also a good idea to then put your whole bag inside one larger, waterproof bag. This gives an extra layer of waterproofing and means you can trap more air before entering the water. This outer layer will also prevent the actual pack from becoming waterlogged.

Tether your pack to your wrist using a quick-release knot so it is easy to detach if needed. It's best if the tether is a couple of meters long so you have room to move.

You can hold onto your pack as you swim to use it for buoyancy, or push it in front of you while using the aggressive stroke. If the pack gets waterlogged, let it go so you can swim and then pull it to shore by the tether.

Related Chapters:

- Freestyle
- Improvised Flotation Aids
- Waterproofing Your Pack

OTHER BODIES OF WATER

Besides rivers, lakes, and oceans, there are other types of water bodies that you may come across. These include bogs, swamps, quicksand, quagmires, and more.

Do not try to walk across them. Lifting your feet while standing will make you sink further. Go around them, or build an improvised bridge using logs, branches, or whatever is around. If this is not viable, there are other methods you can use.

Bogs and Swamps

You can cross a bog or swamp by lying face down with your arms and legs spread. Use a flotation device and slowly swim/pull yourself along. Keep your body horizontal.

Quicksand

Quicksand is a mixture of fine sand (or silt or clay) and water. It has a spongy texture. It's impossible to be completely submerged in quicksand, but you will get stuck. Carrying a pole will help you get out.

When you fall in, remain calm and move slowly. The more you struggle, the more stuck you will get.

Lay your pole on the surface of the quicksand and use it to guide your back into a floating position, with your arms and legs spread out. Shift the pole under your hips, at a right angle to your spine.

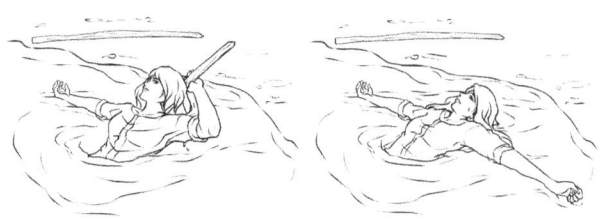

Pull your legs out, one after the other, and move to the nearest solid ground. You can do this without a pole, but it will take longer. The main thing is to move slowly into a horizontal position.

Pulling someone out of quicksand is very difficult. Use a long stick or rope, and do it slowly.

Dense Vegetation

When swimming in dense vegetation, stay near the surface. Thrashing about will get you in trouble. Use a gentle breaststroke and peel away the vegetation around you as you pass through.

Mangrove Swamps

Mangrove swamps are usually found along tropical coastlines. They are best crossed during low tide.

If you're inland trying to get to the ocean, you can work your way through a narrow grove of trees. When you're trying to get inland, you're better off going to the small watercourses (streams or channels).

Always be on the lookout for crocodiles. If you see one, leave the water and get over the mangrove roots.

If the amount of water in the swamp allows it, build a raft.

Back Bays

Back bays are muddy islands found behind the dunes near the ocean. They are very tiring to cross. If you must do so, it's better to find the deep-water sections so you can swim as opposed to trekking through the soft mud. Failing that, look for firmer terrain such as sand, shell, or stone. Trying to cross over the muddy islands is a bad idea, as they're usually too soft.

WATER RESCUE

This section covers essential water rescue skills of others in both pools and open water.

Most of the information in this section mimics professional lifeguard techniques, but it is NOT a replacement for professional lifeguard training! It's for use in emergency situations when no lifeguards are present—for example, if you're hosting a gathering near a lake or pool.

WHEN YOU SEE SOMEONE IN TROUBLE

Anyone can use the following steps if they see someone who needs help in the water. These are simple steps that you can teach your friends and family, including children:

- Keep calm. A person who panics cannot think clearly.
- Shout for help as loudly as you can.
- Ask everyone else to clear the area.
- Ensure there will be no immediate danger to you (from animals, electricity, fire, etc.) while you're attempting the rescue.
- Use land-based rescue techniques in the order given.
- If you cannot perform a land-based rescue, call the emergency services.

Important note: Unless you're trained in water rescue, never enter the water to try and save a victim. A drowning victim can pull you down with him. Even when you are trained, entering the water is a last resort.

SITUATIONAL ASSESSMENT

A situational assessment is a logical process for gathering information and planning based on that information.

The 10:20 System

When you're responsible for the well-being of others near water, you can use the 10:20 system. It's a good way to oversee a designated area.

The 10 stands for 10 seconds. You scan the designated area (e.g., a pool) from one side to the other in 10 seconds. The 20 means that you should be no more than 20 seconds away from getting to any swimmer in your area.

Casualty Priorities and Recognition

The general rule of thumb is to rescue those making the least noise first and the unconscious last.

The four types of casualties, in order of rescue priority, are as follows:

1. **Conscious non-swimmers.** Unable to swim and usually vertical in the water. They may grab hold and drag you down.
2. **Conscious weak swimmers.** Can swim, but are either exhausted or in some other distress. Usually in a forward position attempting to swim. Often co-operative in a rescue.
3. **Conscious injured swimmers.** Can usually keep themselves afloat, but have an injury that they may or may not tell you about. They could be holding their injury. Be careful of the injury while performing a rescue.
4. **Unconscious swimmers.** Often floating motionless and face down in the water, but can be at any depth.

You should rescue the unconscious victim last because they may already be a lost cause. You do not want to waste time that you could spend rescuing a victim with a higher chance of survival.

Recognizing a Distressed Swimmer

A distressed swimmer is any conscious swimmer who is having trouble in the water. If he does not find safety, he can become an unconscious swimmer. You must learn how to recognize a distressed swimmer, so you can rescue him before it is too late.

There are two basic types of swimmers in distress: non-panicking or panicking.

The non-panicking casualty knows he needs help to get to safety. He will be trying to communicate this to you.

A panicking casualty is likely to already be in the drowning phase. He will be thrashing around trying to keep afloat. He may be trying to communicate (either silently or noisily), but the communication will be ineffective.

Making a Plan

It's very important to create a plan of rescue instead of acting straight away. The human brain can process a lot of information at great speed, even in high-stress situations. Once you recognize a casualty, it will only take a couple of seconds for you to assess the situation. This will keep you safe and will also give the victim the best chance of survival.

The first thing you should look for is possible danger. Why is the victim in trouble in the first place? Is the danger still there?

Next, consider your victim's profile. Is he big, small, an adult, a child, unconscious, panicked, injured, etc.?

Finally, what rescue equipment do you have, and/or what can you improvise?

Use the information you gather and the knowledge of your own abilities to decide the best form of rescue.

Due to the endless possibilities of these scenarios, you'll need to be very flexible. For example, should you take the time to find a rescue aid? If so, which rescue aid is best for the situation?

LAND-BASED RESCUES

Land-based rescue techniques are safe to use by almost anyone. Here, they're presented in escalating order. Only use the second one if the first doesn't work, and so on.

GENERAL LAND-BASED RESCUES

In every rescue, watch the victim as much as possible while you're preparing. That way, if he goes under, you can tell others the best place to look. If a second person is present, have him watch the victim while you find equipment and/or help.

Shout and Signal

Your victim may be in a panic. Sometimes, giving simple instructions will be enough for him to save himself. Get his attentional by waving and shouting. Then, in a loud, clear voice, tell him to kick his legs and push towards you or the nearest safe spot (the water's edge, shallow water, etc.).

Throw Rescue

Look for something the victim can use to float on, and throw it to him. The object must be small enough for you to throw, but buoyant enough for the casualty to use as a float, such as a large plastic bottle.

Aim it so the victim can reach it, but do not hit him in the head. Allow for wind and current and aim upstream from the victim. Once he has the object, tell him how to paddle to safety. Unless it presents more danger, he should swim with the current.

Tossing a rope is also considered a throw rescue.

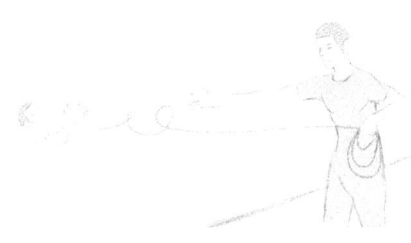

Throw one end of the rope to the victim, and then help to pull him to safety. Stay at least a meter back from the water's edge to prevent you from falling or getting pulled in.

Reach Rescue

Find something that you can hold out to the victim with from dry land, like a stick. Lie down at the edge of the water while reaching out. If possible, hold onto something as well. Lying down and holding onto something prevents the victim from pulling you in.

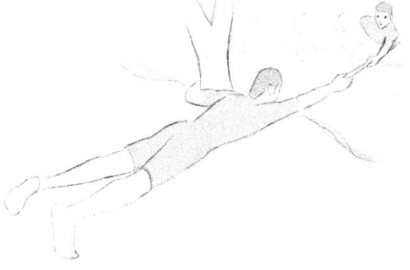

WATER-BASED RESCUES

Only use water-based rescues if land-based rescues are not possible. Like land-based rescues, water-based rescues have a preferred order of use. Here they are in that order.

GENERAL WATER-BASED RESCUES

These first three rescues are far less dangerous than tow rescues, since you avoid direct contact with the victim.

Wading Rescue

A wading rescue is good in water no more than waist deep. Any more than that, and it turns into a towing rescue. The victim must be conscious for this method to work.

Find a rescue aid and enter the water as close to the victim as you can while keeping safe and out of his reach. If possible, keep hold of something on shore. Instruct the victim to grab onto the aid, and pull him to safety.

Boat Rescue

When there is a boat nearby and you know how to use it, you can use a boat rescue. As a rule, avoid bringing the victim on board the boat.

If the victim is unconscious, it's best to have a second rescuer hold his head above water as you drag him to safety. A solo rescuer will have to bring him on board. Be careful not to capsize the boat as you do so.

If the victim is conscious, throw him a tow rope or a float. If he is calm, he can even hold onto the boat, although this is risky with a panicking victim.

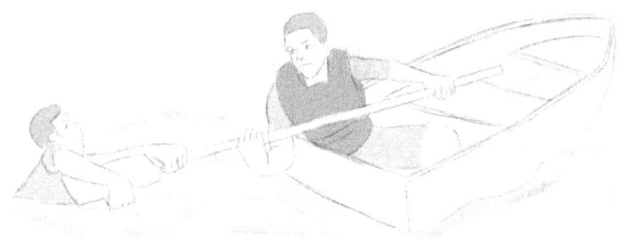

There are many situations where you will have to bring the victim on board—if there's something dangerous in the water or when the distance to land is long, for example. Remember to be flexible.

Swim with an Aid

This is the same as a wading rescue, except you swim the rescue aid to the victim instead of wading. It is useful for conscious victims in deeper waters.

Swimming while holding an aid requires prior practice. Practice taking off your clothes while in the water as well. You can use them as an improvised rescue aid if you are already in the water when someone needs help.

As with a wading rescue, be sure to stay out of the victim's reach. Using the aid is much safer. Help drag him to safety and make sure you are stable before helping him onto land.

Related Chapters:

- Wading

TOWING

Towing is when you have to grab the victim and bring him to safety. This may be for an unconscious victim, because you have no aid, or because the person is too panicked to grab your aid. The latter type of victim is the most dangerous, as they may drag you under the water.

There are several types of rescue tows and the one you use will depend on the specific scenario.

Whenever you approach any victim for a tow, stop a few meters back from him first. Reassess the situation and calm the patient from a safe distance. Assuming he is conscious, tell him what you plan to do and that he should stay calm throughout the process. Continue to reassure him until he is safe on shore.

Armpit Tows

The armpit tow is useful with a co-operative or unconscious victim. It allows you to approach from behind, which is the safest position for you. There are two types of armpit tows, single and double. The one you use depends on what you prefer and the situation at hand.

To do an armpit tow, you must first level the victim off. This is so you can keep his face out of the water and his airway clear. It also places the victim in a horizontal position in the water, making it easier for you to take him to safety.

For the single-armpit tow, approach the victim from behind and grab his armpit with the hand that's one the same side (grab his right armpit with your right hand, for example). Place the elbow of your other arm in the center of his back. Pull with your hand as you push with your elbow. At the same time, use a scissor kick to level him out, face up. Your other hand can assist in the process if needed.

While keeping hold of his armpit, start swimming, so that you drag him in the direction you want to go. Sidestroke works well. Allow your arm to extend until you start to pull him.

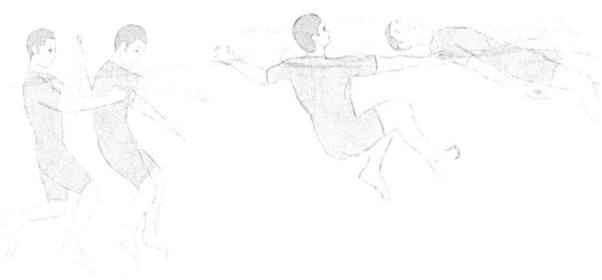

When the victim is larger than you, the double-armpit tow may be easier to use, especially to level him off. Approach the victim from behind and grab both his armpits. Grab his right armpit with your right hand and his left armpit with your left hand. Place both your elbows on his back, and pull with your hands as you push with your elbows. As you do this, use an inverted breaststroke (like in survival backstroke) to help pull him flat on his back. He will now be level.

Continue to kick until your arms lock straight and you start to pull him. You will need to use a continuous and strong kick to keep your victim's face out of the water.

Using the double-armpit tow long-distance is hard, since you have no arms to assist with swimming. A good idea is to start with the double-armpit tow and then switch to the single armpit tow once you have momentum.

You can make the double-armpit tow easier with a flotation aid. Place any long, thin, buoyant object between you and your victim and then tow him as normal. A pool noodle or a rolled-up sleeping mat work well. If possible, swim up with it in place—that is, across your chest and under your armpits.

You may find it more difficult to level the victim when you're using an aid this way. You will need to experiment to see what works best for you. You may even choose to skip the leveling.

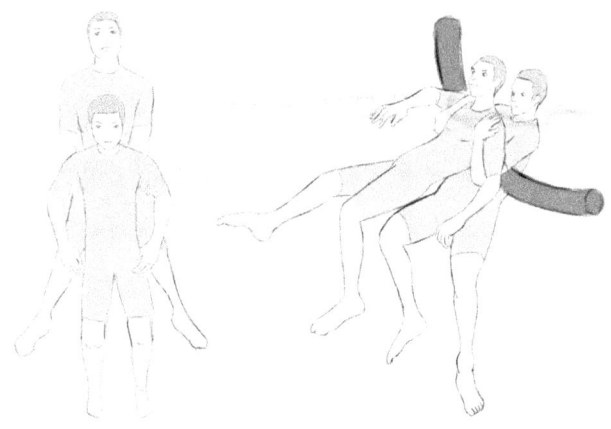

Once you have some momentum, you may be able to free up one of your hands to help you swim.

Every flotation device will act a little differently. Experiment with various options, and especially with things you're likely to have at hand.

Cross Chest Carry

Use the cross-chest carry when rescuing a victim in heavy surf. It's more tiring than other rescues.

Approach the victim from behind and level him off (as described in the armpit-tow instructions). Encircle his chest with one arm. You can place your other hand on his side to help move him into a secure position.

Once you get a good grip, use sidestroke to swim him to safety. Your hip on his back will help to support him. If the victim struggles, you can either tighten your grip or use a defense technique (next chapter).

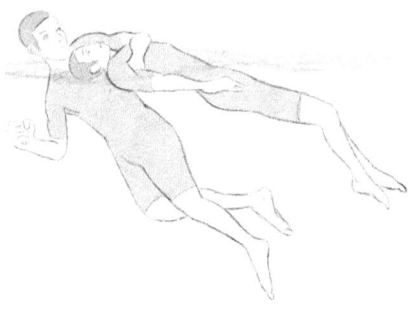

Vice Grip Rollover and Tow

When you suspect your victim has a spinal injury, use the vise-grip rollover and tow.

The vice-grip rollover and tow allow you to turn a facedown victim over and tow him, while protecting his spine. You can also provide rescue breaths to an unconscious victim while towing him. You may wish to do this if the distance to shore is further than you are willing to wait to perform CPR.

To do the rollover, you need to be in water deep enough to allow you to submerge the victim. Grip his jaw with one hand and align your forearm along his sternum.

Place your other hand on the back of the victim's head and align your other forearm along his spine. Squeeze your elbows together. Grip his head, neck, and spine between your forearms.

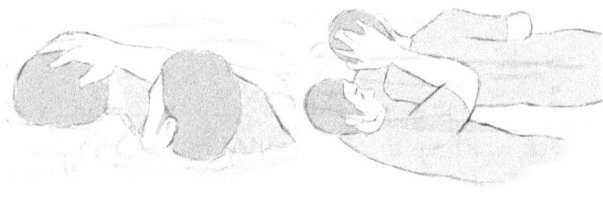

Move forward to level him off. While keeping him as level and stable as you can, roll under him to turn him over. Maintain your vise grip and use a scissor kick to swim.

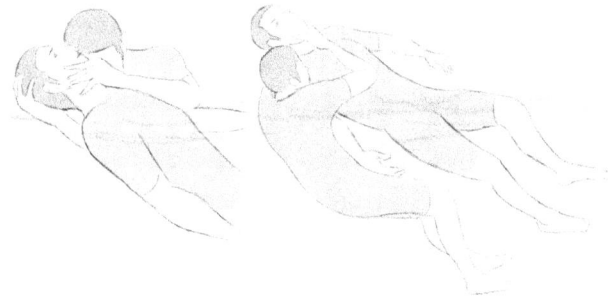

Giving rescue breaths is challenging, but you can do it if the victim is not too big for you. Change your hand on his chin to a pistol grip and lean over to give the breaths.

Note: Giving rescue breaths will compromise the spinal support.

Related Chapters:

- Survival Backstroke

DEFENSE AGAINST A DROWNING VICTIM

A drowning victim can be dangerous to anyone that gets within arm's reach of him. He can grab and pull you down with extreme strength (due to his increased adrenalin) in an effort to save himself. This is why you should only use a tow rescue as a last resort, especially with a panicking victim.

In this chapter, you'll learn how to defend yourself against these "attacks." Practice them on land first, and then in the water. You want to be able to do them instinctively.

Hold-escape techniques in the water are different than normal self-defense techniques. They take the water into account and are non-violent, because the victim does not intend to harm you. His instinct for survival simply overrides his ability to see the negative effects. Defend yourself and then help him, if possible.

General Defense

Whenever a casualty tries to grab you, or as soon as you escape his grip, treat him as an obstruction. Adopt the defensive position by lying on your back with your feet pointed towards him. Kick your legs with the aim of making a big splash. Be careful not to kick the victim.

Kicking your legs does a few things:

- Creates distance.
- Communicates to the victim to not grab you.
- Breaks the victim's grip if he grabs your legs.

When you're grabbed, there are some universal things you can do to escape without harming the victim.

- Press your chin to your chest, raise your shoulders, and cross your arms over your face. This prevents the victim grabbing you around your neck.
- Pull his finger or toe to loosen his grip.
- Poke his armpit.
- Take a big breath and submerge yourself. All releases are more effective when done underwater. Your victim will want to stay above water, so if you go under, he's likely to let you go. At the very least, he will loosen his grip, which will make your escape easier.

The following techniques will let you escape the most common drowning-victim holds. With these and the introductory information given, you can adapt to other situations.

Block

The block is a good preventative technique to use when the victim lunges at you as you approach him from the front. As he lunges, place your open palm against his upper chest.

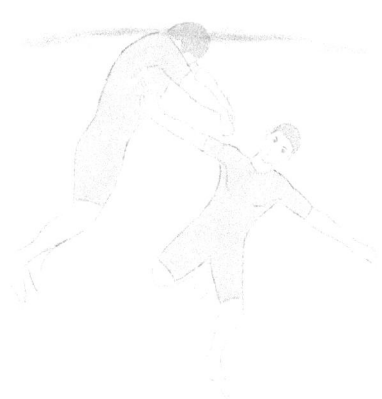

Lean back and submerge, keeping your arm(s) extended as you do so. Swim away while you're underwater, and resurface at a safe distance from him.

Wrist/Arm-Grab Escape

When you're grabbed by your arm or wrist, reach across with your free hand and push down on your victim's shoulder. Kick upward at the same time.

While maintaining downward pressure on his shoulder, jerk up hard with your trapped arm. Repeat this until you are free.

Release the victim and swim back to a safe distance.

Head-Hold Escape

Use this technique when the victim grabs you around your head and neck from either the front or back.

Protect your throat by taking a quick breath and tucking your chin into your shoulder. Clap your hands above your head a few times so that you submerge underwater. This will also drag the victim underwater, which will often encourage him to let you go.

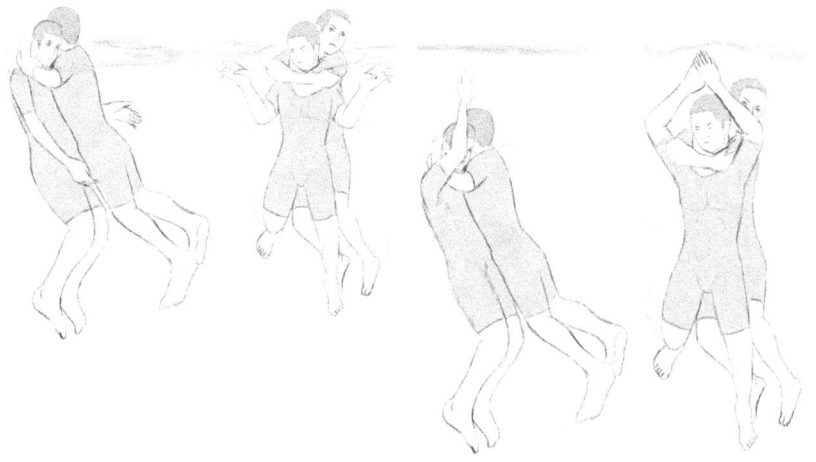

Apply an upward grab and thrust with your thumbs on his brachial pressure points. Find these on the inside of his upper arm, a little above his elbow.

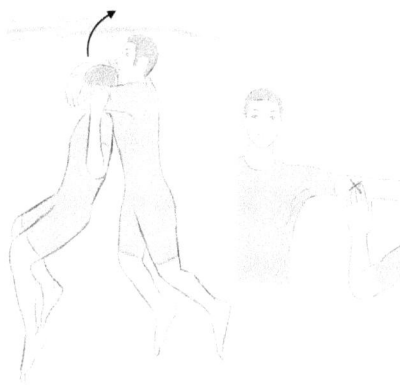

Swim away while you are underwater, and resurface at a safe distance from him.

ROPE RESCUES

These rescues assume you only have one rope (such as a throw bag) and no other specialist equipment. Using this minimalist approach leaves you with the simplest of rope rescue techniques.

If you enjoy whitewater sports, you should be carrying more equipment. Take a professional course on how to use it.

Be sure to review the Throwing Rope chapter before training in these rope rescues. It is in the River Crossings section, under the heading Rope Crossings.

If you have the manpower, place safety rescuers for all rope rescues. Put one upstream from the rescue to warn and redirect or stop anyone coming down the river. Place one or more safety rescuers downstream from the rescue as well. This is in case a rescuer becomes a victim (if he falls in the water, for example). It also ensures that if the first rescue fails, there will be an immediate backup.

Note: Safety rescuers are not drawn in most of the following demonstration pictures.

LAND-BASED ROPE RESCUES

Entering water is always more dangerous than performing a land-based rescue. In the case of swift water, the danger of a water-based rescue increases. Use a land-based rope rescue if possible.

Pendulum Rescue

The general idea of a pendulum rescue is to throw a rope to the victim so he can grab onto it as he drifts by. He will then swing to shore in an arc, like a pendulum.

The pendulum rescue is fast to deploy but a couple of things can go wrong.

- The victim may miss the rope.
- If the rescuer is not well anchored, he may get pulled into the water.

To do a pendulum rescue, you must position yourself downstream from the victim. Be sure to give yourself enough time to deploy the rope. Anchor yourself if needed, depending on the weight of the victim and the force of the current. It's a good idea to hold onto a tree or have a second rescuer hold onto you.

You should also consider what obstacles the victim may swing into because of your position.

Throw the rope a little in front of and past the victim, so that he can grab it as he floats past in the defensive position.

Instruct the victim to grab hold of the line and place it over his shoulder. This will orient his head towards the rescuer. He must stay on his back. Keep stationary and allow the current to swing the victim towards the shore. Once the pendulum effect has finished, pull the victim the rest of the way.

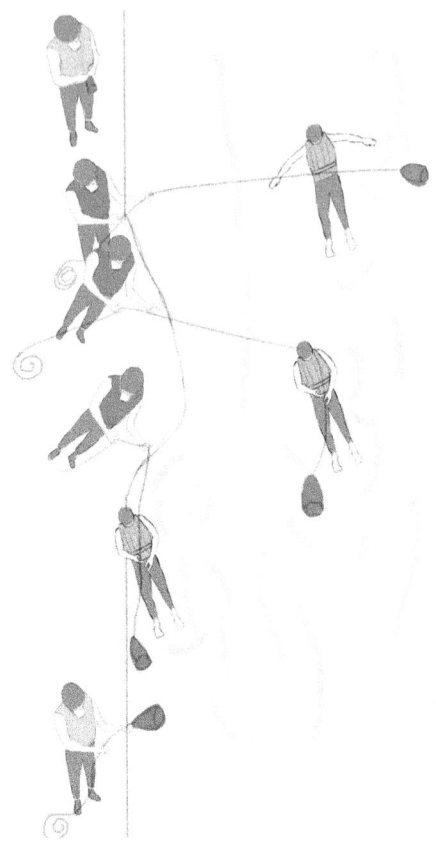

To counteract the victim's weight, use a belay position by passing the rope around the upper bit of your butt. For extra stability, you can sit on it, and if you have the manpower, you can have someone help hold you down.

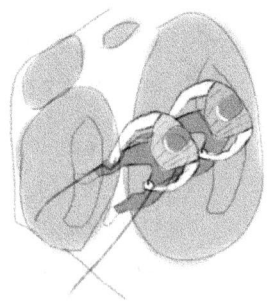

If it's possible (and not dangerous), take a few steps back inland after you've thrown the rope. This will increase the pendulum effect, as well as reduce the load you need to bear. Let out some of the rope as you get repositioned. Once you're stable, pull the rope tight to start the pendulum.

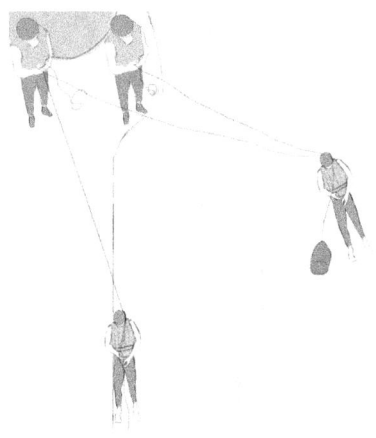

Stabilization Line

A stabilization line is a rope you fix across the river to catch the victim. It takes more time to set up, but lessens the chances of missing the catch.

It's also useful for providing a general support line the victim can use to hold his head above water. This can be a lifesaver in cases such as a foot entrapment when the current is forcing the victim down.

The stabilization line generally requires at least two people, one on either side of the river. You could do it with one person by tying one or both ends to something, but you would have to cross the river.

The smaller the angle between the rescuer(s) and the victim, the easier it will on the rescuers.

Once the victim catches the line, he can pull himself to safety.

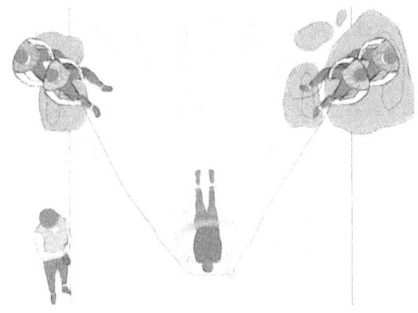

Kiwi Cinch

The Kiwi Cinch is the only simple land-based rescue you can use with an unconscious victim. It requires the victim to be drifting close to shore.

Do it by looping the rope around the victim and then pulling him in.

As with stabilization line, it is possible to do the Kiwi Cinch with one person, but it's much easier with two. This demonstration uses two people.

Each rescuer coils one half of the rope from the center out. This way, they have the same length of rope.

As the victim drifts past, the rescuers throw the rope around him in a big loop. The two rescuers must communicate well, so that they throw their ends of the rope at the same time. They must hold onto the other end of the rope.

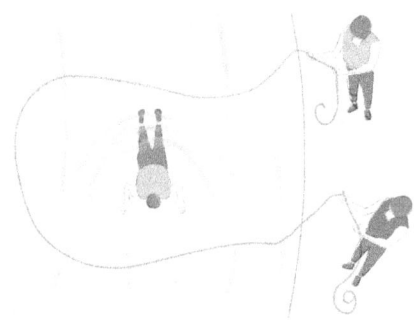

They must then cross the rope to create a closed loop around the victim. To do this, the two rescuers must swap places. The upstream rescuer walks behind the downstream rescuer. His rope will cross on top. The downstream rescuer moves up at the same time.

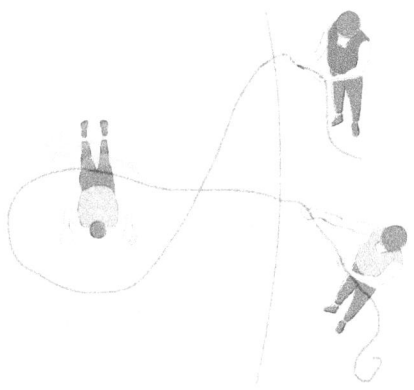

Once the two are in place, they tighten the loop (the cinch) around the victim, preferably around his torso. The new upstream rescuer anchors himself in a sitting belay. The downstream rescuer pulls his side of the rope to swing the victim to shore.

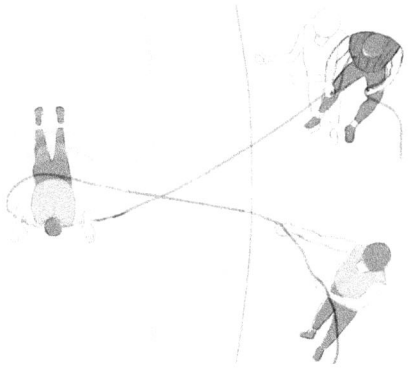

SWIMMING ROPE RESCUES

Swimming rope rescues need the rescuer to enter the water to save the victim. This includes wading. Use them for unconscious victims, floating equipment, or anything that can't self-rescue.

Simple Rope Tether

With the simple rope tether, attach the rescuer to a rope as he wades out to rescue the victim. Secure the other end of the rope on shore by tying it to something or having a second rescuer as a belayer.

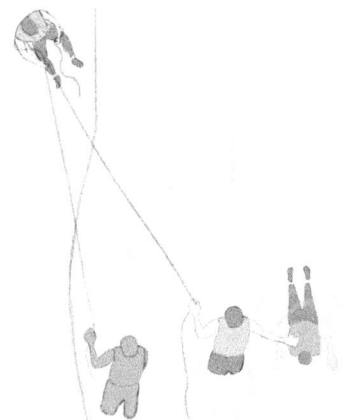

Tethered Swimmer

The tethered swimmer rescue is when the rescuer swims up to the victim instead of wading. The rescuer will need two hands, so tie him to the tether.

Although a tied belay would work, it's best if the belayer is human, as he can then feed out the line as needed, as well as help pull the rescuer and victim to shore. The belayer should feed the rope loosely, so that the swimmer isn't held back by it.

If the victim is wearing something on his upper body (such as a life jacket) the rescuer can grab onto it. If not, they should use an armpit tow. If there's a human rescuer on shore, he can swing or pull the rescuer and victim to shore. If not, they can drift downstream until the line gets taut. They will then swing towards shore.

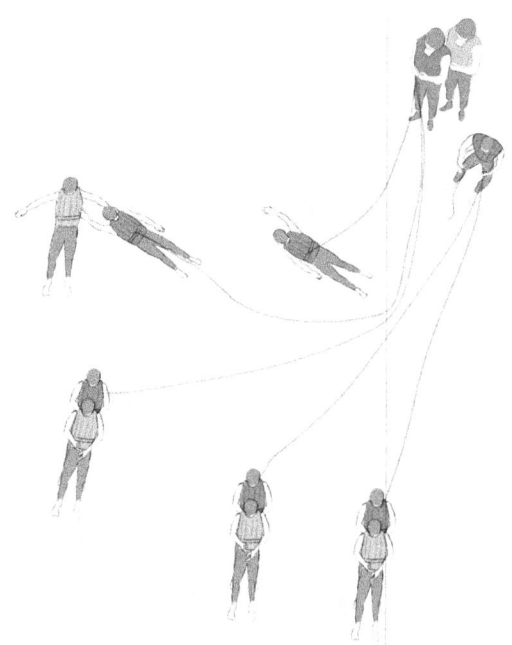

Related Chapters:

- Wading

THANKS FOR READING

Dear reader,

Thank you for reading *Survival Swimming*.

If you enjoyed this book, please leave a review where you bought it. It helps more than most people think.

Get The Survival Fitness Plan App

It's like having Sam Fury as a personal coach to train you in the Survival Fitness Plan whenever you want!

Download it FREE at:

https://www.survivalfitnessplan.com/app

Thanks again for your support.

REFERENCES

Courtley, C. (2012). *SEAL Survival Guide: A Navy SEAL's Secrets to Surviving Any Disaster.* Gallery Books.

Ferrero, F. (2009). *Whitewater Safety and Rescue: Essential Knowledge For Canoeists, Kayakers, And Raft Guides.* Falcon Guides.

Laughlin, T. (2004). *Total Immersion: The Revolutionary Way To Swim Better, Faster, and Easier.* Touchstone.\Mann, D. Pezzulo, R. (2012). *The U.S. Navy SEAL Survival Handbook: Learn the Survival Techniques and Strategies of America's Elite Warriors.* Skyhorse Publishing.

Smith, S. (2013). *The Navy SEAL Weight Training Workout: The Complete Guide to Navy SEAL Fitness - Phase 2 Program.* Hatherleigh Press.

Sunmacher, W. Walbridge, C. (1995). *Whitewater Rescue Manual: New Techniques for Canoeists, Kayakers, and Rafters.* International Marine/Ragged Mountain Press.

Treinish, S. (2017). *Water Rescue: Principles and Practice to NFPA 1006 and 1670.* Jones & Bartlett Learning.

Wiseman, J. (2015). *SAS Survival Guide.* William Collins.

Young, M. (2016). *The Complete Beginners Guide To Swimming: Professional guidance and support to help you through every stage of learning how to swim.* Educate and Learn Publishing.

ABOUT THE SURVIVAL FITNESS PLAN

When in danger, you have two options: fight or flight.

The Survival Fitness Plan focuses on training in the best methods of flight and fight as a form of exercise. Skills covered include:

Self-Defense. SFP Self-Defense is an efficient and effective form of self-defense derived from a wide range of street-effective martial arts.

Parkour. Training in SFP Parkour will teach you how cross terrain on foot with maximum speed and efficiency while still overcoming obstacles in the safest way possible.

Swimming. Learn to swim for endurance and/or speed using the most efficient strokes there are.

Mountain Bike Riding. Discover the skills and techniques you need to go as fast as you can over uncertain terrain in the safest way possible on a bike.

Health and Fitness. General health and fitness including body conditioning, nutrition, and meditation.

ABOUT SAM FURY

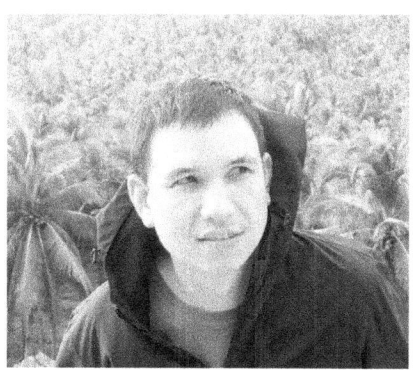

Sam Fury has had a passion for survival, evasion, resistance, and escape (SERE) training since he was a young boy growing up in Australia.

This led him to years of training and career experience in related subjects, including martial arts, military training, survival skills, outdoor sports, and sustainable living.

These days, Sam spends his time refining existing skills, gaining new skills, and sharing what he learns via the Survival Fitness Plan website.

www.SurvivalFitnessPlan.com

- amazon.com/author/samfury
- goodreads.com/SamFury
- facebook.com/SamFuryOfficial
- instagram.com/SamFuryOfficial
- youtube.com/SurvivalFitnessPlan